NURSING – ISSUES, PROBLEMS, AND CHALLENGES SERIES

PSYCHIATRIC NURSES PERCEPTIONS OF THE CONSTITUENTS OF THE THERAPEUTIC RELATIONSHIP

NURSING – ISSUES, PROBLEMS, AND CHALLENGES SERIES

Psychiatric Nurses Perceptions of the Constituents of the Therapeutic Relationship
Adrian Scanlon
2010 ISBN: 978-1-60876-365-8

NURSING – ISSUES, PROBLEMS, AND CHALLENGES SERIES

PSYCHIATRIC NURSES PERCEPTIONS OF THE CONSTITUENTS OF THE THERAPEUTIC RELATIONSHIP

ADRIAN SCANLON

Nova Science Publishers, Inc.
New York

Copyright © 2010 by Nova Science Publishers, Inc.

All rights reserved. No part of this book may be reproduced, stored in a retrieval system or transmitted in any form or by any means: electronic, electrostatic, magnetic, tape, mechanical photocopying, recording or otherwise without the written permission of the Publisher.

For permission to use material from this book please contact us:
Telephone 631-231-7269; Fax 631-231-8175
Web Site: http://www.novapublishers.com

NOTICE TO THE READER

The Publisher has taken reasonable care in the preparation of this book, but makes no expressed or implied warranty of any kind and assumes no responsibility for any errors or omissions. No liability is assumed for incidental or consequential damages in connection with or arising out of information contained in this book. The Publisher shall not be liable for any special, consequential, or exemplary damages resulting, in whole or in part, from the readers' use of, or reliance upon, this material.

Independent verification should be sought for any data, advice or recommendations contained in this book. In addition, no responsibility is assumed by the publisher for any injury and/or damage to persons or property arising from any methods, products, instructions, ideas or otherwise contained in this publication.

This publication is designed to provide accurate and authoritative information with regard to the subject matter covered herein. It is sold with the clear understanding that the Publisher is not engaged in rendering legal or any other professional services. If legal or any other expert assistance is required, the services of a competent person should be sought. FROM A DECLARATION OF PARTICIPANTS JOINTLY ADOPTED BY A COMMITTEE OF THE AMERICAN BAR ASSOCIATION AND A COMMITTEE OF PUBLISHERS.

LIBRARY OF CONGRESS CATALOGING-IN-PUBLICATION DATA

Scanlon, Adrian.
  Psychiatric nurses perceptions of the constituents of the therapeutic relationship / Adrian Scanlon.
       p. ; cm.
  Includes bibliographical references and index.
  ISBN 978-1-60876-365-8 (softcover)
  1. Psychiatric nursing. 2. Nurse and patient. 3. Therapeutic alliance. I. Title.
  [DNLM: 1. Mental Disorders--nursing. 2. Nurse-Patient Relations. 3. Nursing Theory. 4. Psychiatric Nursing. 5. Research Design. WY 160 S283p 2009], RC440.S3312 2009
     616.89'0231--dc22,   2009037456

Published by Nova Science Publishers, Inc. ✣ New York

CONTENTS

Preface		vii
Introduction		ix
Chapter One	Background to the Literature	1
Chapter Two	The Study Design	19
Chapter Three	Findings	39
Chapter Four	Discussion	67
Conclusion		79
Appendix One	Map of Counseling	81
Appendix Two	Grounded Theory Process	83
Appendix Three	Research Questions/Topic Guide	85
Appendix Four	Informed Consent Form - Therapeutic Relationship Research	87
Appendix Five	Ethical Approval Letter	89
Appendix Six	GANT Chart	91
Appendix Seven	Resources and Study Management	93
Appendix Eight	Reply from the Director of Nursing	95
Appendix Nine	Open Coding - Participant 1	97

Appendix Ten Interview Notes 103

Appendix Eleven Audit Trail 113

Appendix Twelve Feedback from Psychiatric Nurses and Participants in
Relation to the Findings 119

Index 121

PREFACE

Psychiatric nursing is invariably linked with a therapeutic role; however the question remains unanswered in relation to the extent psychiatric nurses perceive the importance of the constituents of the therapeutic relationship. The aim of this research is to ascertain the nature and comprehension psychiatric nurses assign this therapeutic role. The subject relates significantly to the role of the psychiatric nurses in relation to awareness of elements of the therapeutic relationship in his or her practice and the understanding and identifying this role clearly and unambiguously.

Grounded theory methodology was utilized to develop these conceptualizations to elicit a theory relating to what comprises the therapeutic relationship. Semi-structured depth interviews were conducted with 6 generic registered psychiatric nurses who have between two and ten years of experience.

The objective of the research was to formulate a theory relating to constituents of the therapeutic relationship to inform professional psychiatric nursing practice and to provide a theoretical framework to inform conscious psychiatric nursing practice in relation to forming therapeutic relationships. Strauss and Corbin (1990) describe one of the purposes of research is to guide practitioners' practices and to develop a basic knowledge. The aim of this research was to fulfill this purpose; building theory implies interpreting data that must be conceptualized and the concepts related to a view of reality.

The main findings of the research related to how psychiatric nurses learn to form these relationships and what skills are utilized within the relationship. The research discovered that the therapeutic relationship is therapeutic, but the degree of positive change is difficult to measure. The study also highlighted that the learning that takes place in relation to the development of therapeutic relationships is an experiential process and begs the question; is the focus of psychiatric nurse training, in relation to the therapeutic relationship, located appropriately?

INTRODUCTION

This chapter begins with an overview of the research question and how this question is informed by previous practice. The question is contextualized by the historical influences on psychiatric nursing practice in relation to formation of therapeutic relationships and synthesizing this with contemporary psychiatric nursing. The significance to psychiatric nursing practice and purpose of the research are also identified. Definitions of important terms used in the course of the study are made explicit.

The Research Problem

The growing emphasis on nurses to provide evidence to support best practice has been a major impetus for study in all areas of nursing. Psychiatric nursing, although advanced in areas of interpersonal skills and manpower management, have been sadly lacking in the area of research relating to practice. This study aims to provide empirical evidence in relation to understanding a fundamental aspect of the psychiatric nurses' role, namely what constitutes the therapeutic relationship.

While a positive therapeutic relationship is a necessary pre-requisite for a successful therapeutic outcome, it remains a largely unmeasured phenomenon that is not well understood. A review of the theoretical and empirical literature indicates that the elements of the therapeutic relationship in relation to interactive, subjective, dynamic components have been largely ignored (LM. Weibe, University of Toronto, Toronto, unpublished dissertation).

This study aims to explore the research in relation to the components of the therapeutic relationship elicited in the literature. Whilst this is of significance, I will attempt to bracket this knowledge and form a theory from the information provided by the participants. Psychiatric nurses intuitively form relationships with patients and these relationships invariably are stated to be therapeutic. Exploration of this phenomenon in a scientific sense is fundamental to understanding how and why psychiatric nurses perform his or her role. The early work of Peplau (1952) has acted as a catalyst for further study in this area and developments to advance psychiatric nursing practice have been significant. This study is designed to add to the growing evidence to promote conscious competence in psychiatric nursing.

BACKGROUND TO THE RESEARCH PROBLEM

Psychiatric nursing can be seen as occupying two care domains as indicated by the role or title; to nurse implies a doing activity and psychiatric nursing involves a competence and knowledge of conditions within the spectrum of the study and treatment of mental diseases (Rolfe, 1990). The role and function of mental health nurses has evolved from the custodial attendant to the inquiring professional practitioner. This evolution has necessitated a fundamental shift from assisting medics in the care of inmates to autonomous therapeutic change agents (Chambers, 1998).

Fundamental to any research inquiry involving the discipline of psychiatry is the appreciation of the complexity and convoluted concept of the psyche or mind. Medical and natural sciences dominate medical practice and have influenced scientific inquiry in psychiatric nursing. Psychiatric nursing however has developed scientific respectability in its own right, as illustrated by Peplau (1952) who was one of the first scholars to locate psychiatric nursing within the American Neo-Freudian tradition of theorists. Contemporary psychiatric nursing therefore is based on the notion that therapeutic relationships are concerned with reactions of human beings to mental distress and illness and how individuals are assisted to cope or adapt to life experiences (Chambers, 1998).

The fact that psychiatric nursing and psychiatry is complex per se is reflected in the complexity of questions that are addressed by research, these questions are informed by human experiences of the psyche and outcomes are not easily measured and are epistemologically difficult to locate. Omery et al (1995) stated that when answering questions relating to human experiences nurses need to be assured in asserting the utilization of less favored research methodologies to refine, advance knowledge and understanding to improve the quality of care delivery. In this sense qualitative and naturalistic methods that are appropriate methods for certain research questions, are the appropriate approach to research the psychiatric nurses' experiences of the constituent of the therapeutic relationship.

The literature seems to indicate two observations relating to psychiatric nursing knowledge; one proposes a biological basis of mental illness (Gournay, 1996), the second is a humanistic view concerned with social determinants of mental illness and the subsequent relationship with the nurse (Barker et al, 1995). The approach of Humanistic Existentialism with a dual emphasis on suffering and care is seen as a natural maturational philosophy for the whole of nursing in the future. However with the emphasis on the psychological anguish of the existential dilemma it seems to be particularly suited to mental health nursing (Bevis, 1982). What humanism does do according to Bevis is to make it acceptable for individuals to deviate from these scientific norms and so enable the individual to choose about nursing care and medical treatment in accord with their own wishes and personal judgment. This fundamental shift enables nursing to move beyond the restrictions of practicing within the medical model.

The purpose of this study is to provide empirical evidence to support a claim that psychiatric nurses fully understand the components of therapeutic relationships. Barker (1998), Chambers (1998), Peplau (1952), Travelbee (1966) testify to the fact that the therapeutic relationship is "the rock" on which psychiatric nursing is built. Therefore a full and unequivocal understanding of what forms these relationships is paramount to performing the role of a psychiatric nurse.

The location of the therapeutic relationship within the role of psychiatric nursing therefore, as indicated in the literature, is an illusive concept (Barker, 1998, Gournay, 1996). Peplau (1972) was convinced of the centrality of this interpersonal and psychotherapeutic aspect in nursing. The Expert Review Committee on Psychiatric Nursing further emphasized the shift away from the medico-psychiatric model by highlighting four main areas of nursing: educational, technical, social and interpersonal, of which the interpersonal aspect was central to the task of the nurse (World Health Organization, 1956). Travelbee (1966, 1969) additionally stressed the interpersonal or therapeutic relationship is a fundamental aspect of psychiatric nursing in his seminal works. He illustrated that without the therapeutic relationship psychiatric nursing could not have a therapeutic, healing or change agent role.

Altshul (1972) argued that some psychiatrists viewed psychiatric nurses occupying a therapeutic role as exceeding his or her authority, in a service that continues to be dominated by the medical profession. A personal experience of this author on a psychiatric acute admission unit; overheard a conversation between two psychiatrists and a Director of Nursing, this conversation espoused the virtue of male nurses six foot two tall, well built and able to control patients physically. This conversation did not take place in the 19th century; it took place within the last five years, illustrating clearly where some psychiatrists locate contemporary psychiatric nurses.

Peavy (1996) described the need to determine and explore the paradigm shift from locating the therapeutic relationship within the paradigm of positivism, as being a scientific undertaking; to locating the therapeutic relationship within a culture of healing and describing activities as cultural practices. This shift would not only demystify the location of the therapeutic relationship within psychiatric nursing, it would also sociologically place interpersonal skills and the therapeutic relationship within the discipline of psychiatric nursing. Peavy (1996) argues that when individuals are experiencing pain or despair, some action is warranted either by the individual or by a concerned person; this action is an accepted justification for a therapeutic intervention. He additionally asserts that three essential ingredients have the capacity to support individuals in distress. These ingredients are to clarify aspects of his or her life world, offer hope and encouragement and provide comfort and support.

In addition to the afore mentioned paradigm shift Barker (1998) also proposes new and old paradigms; referring to the old paradigm of essentially rational, analytic, linear, objectifying, fragmenting, dismantling, disempowering and distancing approach of human distress. It is suggested that this paradigm is formed by predominantly masculine values and induces a patriarchal imbalance and fails to acknowledge the feminine values associated with post-modern society. The new paradigm acknowledges the value of balancing masculine and feminine values of post positivist methodology. The methodology and epistemology informing this new paradigm reflects qualitative research methods and this is fundamental to locate human factors within research. This paradigm shift has repercussions for the research of the constituents of the therapeutic relationship. Psychiatric nursing places large emphasis on the reciprocal nature of interpersonal relationships. If the emphasis of the relationship is reciprocal, the relationship from the perspective of the patient would necessitate more involvement and empowerment of mental health users. This increased involvement would enable an increased understanding of patient care issues from the care recipient.

These changing paradigms have initiated a debate in relation to the value of positivist and post positivist methodologies and indeed the rationale to measure mental health nursing interventions. Omery et al (1995) postulated one such aspect of the debate when espousing the notion of the chaos theory. Barker (1998) described the chaos theory as being the answer for researchers who seek a certainty principle to apply to research practice.

Chambers (1998) argues that whatever epistemology or grand theories are utilized to measure humanistic or components associated with interpersonal relationships, within psychiatric nursing, it may be of value to allow for spontaneous reactions between individuals. He argues that for the patients' value is placed on attitudinal and personality traits such as trust, genuineness, warmth and respect.

In addition to philosophical assumptions, theoretical conceptualizations and methodological identification psychiatric nurses are without a doubt professionally socialized to perform his or her role in certain ways. Chambers (1998) made reference to the fact that philosophical beliefs and values espoused by individuals are flavored and influenced by socialization issues. Numerous studies have been conducted in relation to the socialization of nurses indicating that socialization factors are powerful and pervasive (Davies, 1993, Gerrish, 2000, Gray and Smith, 2000, Philpin, 1999). All these scholars conclude that the socialization experiences of nurses affect clinical practice irrespective of educational experiences shaping practice.

THE RESEARCH QUESTION

Having identified the purpose and research problem a number of questions emerge which provide focus and direction to the phenomena under investigation. These questions are formed on a tentative basis that gives a philosophical direction to commence the study. Whilst appreciating that the method of study is dictated by the question and the emerging data influences resultant analysis, constant comparative method engages suitably with, both the question and the philosophical stance. The questions were:

1. How do psychiatric nurses form therapeutic liaisons with patients?
2. How do they differ from any other kind of relationship?
3. What makes therapeutic relationships therapeutic or curative?
4. How do psychiatric nurses learn to form these therapeutic relationships?
5. When do psychiatric nurses learn to form these therapeutic relationships?

SIGNIFICANCE OF THE STUDY

Emphasis continues to be placed on the professionalization of nursing and the necessity for nurses to practice firstly within his or her scope of practice and secondly utilizing evidence based practice (An Bord Altranais, 2000, Hamer and Collinson, 1999). The notion that informs this study and what makes it a significant research endeavor is the questioning of the fundamental role of psychiatric nurses. Namely if psychiatric nurses claim to form therapeutic relationships with patients, are they doing this knowingly, with a complete understanding of why, how and when these relationships are formed? The findings of this study may advance an understanding and formulate a theory of the nature and constituents of the therapeutic relationship. The study may open a debate as to how psychiatric nurses perform their basic roles and how these are learned. A review of the literature indicated a dearth of studies on this particular subject; the findings may therefore advance further study into this fundamental aspect of psychiatric nursing care provision.

Definition of Terms

For the purposes of this study therapeutic relationship refers to the relationship between psychiatric patients and psychiatric nurses. This relationship is stated to be therapeutic; however it is fundamental to the study to determine a difference between this relationship and other life relationships. Therapeutic role refers to some form of intervention on behalf of the psychiatric nurse to induce a positive or curative change by a psychiatric patient.

This chapter began by identifying the research problem, namely the clear unambiguous understanding by psychiatric nurses of what constitutes the therapeutic relationship. A historical perspective was described in an attempt to contextualize a contemporary position. The study question focuses the research on the appropriate usage of therapeutic relationships in psychiatric nursing, whether it is intuitive or learned. The purpose and significance of the study are clearly stated and how the results may be further utilized is stated. An explanation of terms used in the study that the reader may not be familiar with is also defined.

What follows in chapter one is an introduction to relevant literature in the area relating to the therapeutic relationship in psychiatric nursing. The review covers published and unpublished material on the role identification in psychiatric nursing and how this relates to the therapeutic relationship. Related areas such as counseling and psychotherapy in nursing are also examined. Key studies are identified and critically analyzed. The constant comparative method does mean however that the question and the findings will be constantly compared to the knowledge available. Chapter two will describe the research design and how and why the methodology is appropriate for the research question stated. Chapter three will explore in detail the findings of the study. Chapter four will discuss these findings and provide theoretical sensitivity in relation to the phenomenon under investigation, by locating the findings professionally, personally and with the a priori knowledge.

REFERENCES

Altshul A. (1972) A Study of interaction patterns in acute psychiatric wards. Edinburgh, Churchill Livingstone.

An Bord Altranais. (2000) Scope of Nursing and Midwifery Practice Framework. Dublin, An Bord Altranais.

Barker P. (1998) The future of the theory of interpersonal relation? A personal reflection on Peplau's legacy. *Journal of Psychiatric and Mental Health Nursing.* 5, 213-220.

Bevis EO. (1982) Curriculum building in nursing- a process, 3rd edn. St Louis, CV Mosby.

Chambers M. (1998) Interpersonal mental health nursing: Research issues and challenges. *Journal of Psychiatric and Mental Health Nursing.* 5, 203-211.

Davies E. (1993) Clinical role modelling: uncovering hidden knowledge. *Journal of Advanced Nursing.* 18, 4, 627-636.

Gerrish K. (2000) Still fumbling along? A comparative study of the newly qualified nurse's perception of the transition from student to qualified nurse. *Journal of Advanced Nursing.* 32(2), 473-480.

Gournay K. (1996) Schizophrenia: a review of the contemporary literature and implications for mental health nursing theory practice and education. *Journal of Psychiatric and Mental Health Nursing.* 4, 441-446.

Gray M. and Smith L. (2000) the qualities of an effective mentor from the student nurse's perspective: findings from a longitudinal qualitative study. *Journal of Advanced Nursing.* 32, 6, 1542-1549.

Hamer S. and Collinson G. (1999) Achieving evidence based practice: a handbook for practitioners. London, Bailliere Tindall.

Omery A., Kasper CE. and Sage GG. (1995) In search of nursing science. London, Sage Publications.

Peplau HE. (1952) Interpersonal relations in nursing. New York, Putnam.

Peplau HE. (1972) The nurse as counsellor. *Journal of American College Health.* 35, 11-14.

Peavy RV. (1996) Counselling as a culture of healing. *British Journal of Guidance Counselling.* 24(1), 141-150.

Philpin M. (1999) The impact of Project 2000 reforms on the occupational socialisation of nurses. *Journal of Advanced Nursing.* 29(6), 1326-1331.

Rolfe G. (1990) The assessment of therapeutic attitudes in the psychiatric setting. *Journal of Advanced Nursing.* 15, 564-570.

Travelbee J. (1966) Interpersonal aspects of nursing. Philadelphia, F.A. Davis Company.

Travelbee J. (1969) Intervention in psychiatric nursing. Process in the one to one relationship. Philadelphia, F.A. Davis Company.

World Health Organisation. (1956) First report of the expert committee on psychiatric nursing. Geneva, WHO.

Chapter One

BACKGROUND TO THE LITERATURE

The review of the literature begins with a synopsis of the literature search strategy, followed by details of relevant published and unpublished material. Relevant literature related to the examination of meaning assigned to the therapeutic relationship in psychiatric nursing is reviewed. Examination of content and methods utilized to elicit meaning of therapeutic relationship is critically discussed. Whilst the author appreciates the need to review relevant research relating to the subject to situate the study, it is also pertinent to allow the emerging data to determine reality and to produce an informed theory. Commentary by experts in the field of communication, interpersonal skills, counseling and dynamics in human behavior are discussed. Key studies are reviewed in detail including their aims, methodologies, findings and limitations. Any gaps in the knowledge relating to the therapeutic relationship and the understanding of its implementation are also examined. The chapter concludes with a summary of the material reviewed.

REVIEW OF THE LITERATURE IN NATURALISTIC INQUIRY

Positivist research is probably the research most readers would be familiar with and this research process is a linear analytical process that dictates an extensive literature review to ascertain gaps, test hypotheses to contribute ideas to a body of knowledge. In contrast grounded theory research requires not reviewing any of the literature in the area under study. This statement is made in an understanding that the process of theory generation is not contaminated, constrained by, inhibited, stifled or otherwise impeded by influences other than the analysis of data (Glaser, 1992). To quote Glaser (1992 p32) *the researcher should not worry about covering the literature in the same field before his research begins, since it will always be there.* Hutchinson and Wilson (2001) maintain that a literature review is written before data collection and analysis to build a case for the proposed research. The literature review in grounded theory provides context to concepts and an awareness of gaps in the literature. Grounded theorists maintain a second literature review is required to link a priori knowledge and new theory or evidence (Hutchinson and Wilson, 2001).

LITERATURE SEARCH STRATEGY

The literature search involved exploring the published and unpublished material relating to the area of the therapeutic relationship. Most of the literature that was initially located referred to therapeutic relationships in the field of psychology, which although provided interesting reading and relevant, to a point, did not apply specifically to psychiatric nursing. Related areas of counseling, communication and interpersonal relationships were also examined. The searches involved utilization of OVID databases and scanning library catalogues. The databases included Medline, Cinahl, Psychinfo and other health related electronic databases. Keywords used during this exploration of the databases were therapy, therapeutic relationship, psychiatry, psychiatric nursing, nursing and in various combinations of these words.

Initial searches of Medline and Cinahl provided very few empirical studies relating to the area of the therapeutic relationship in psychiatric nursing. The associated area of counseling provided citations, mainly from the 1980s and 1990s, but unfortunately these had more relevance to the field of psychology. The emphasis of this study is psychiatric nursing practice and these studies do not apply to the area under investigation. What was evident during the search was a great deal of commentary, since the 1950s, was in relation to the changing role of the psychiatric nurse. This seems not coincidental with the publication of comment by Peplau (1952), who appears to have ignited this debate. Psychinfo offered more promising research articles related to the phenomena under investigation. These articles seemed to be in two stages of publication. Firstly the 1950s and 1960s and secondly late 1990s to the present, perhaps fuelled by the requirement to practice utilizing evidence based practice.

Although some of these studies were both relevant and provided interesting comment, none of the studies were specific to Irish mental health nursing. This disappointing dearth of empirical evidence is surprising due to the amount of anecdotal literature that is available in relation to interpersonal relationships and interpersonal communication. The search resulted in three significant studies relating to how psychiatric nurses perform their therapeutic role (AC. Berkery, Adelphi University, NY, unpublished dissertation, KJ. Evans, University Microfilms International, Auburn University, AL, unpublished dissertation, LM. Weibe, University of Toronto, Toronto, unpublished dissertation).

A search of libraries in University College Dublin, Waterford Institute of Technology and Waterford Regional Hospital provided a number of texts (Altshul, 1972, Burnard, 1994, Peplau, 1952, Travalbee, 1966). These texts proved to be important works to locate the phenomena under investigation in context. Although most texts are dated they provide seminal commentary by experts. These texts have been re-published on a number of occasions. The material utilized in the literature review were journal articles, both theoretical and empirical sources, fortunately most were available, some were located through inter-library loans and texts borrowed from various locations.

LITERATURE SEARCH-HISTORICAL CONTEXT

The later part of the 19th century saw a slow transition from paternalistic management of patient care, to the utilisation of interpersonal skills, involving the development of change relationships between attendants and inmates. However medical dominance prevailed to restrict the development of therapeutic endeavours. The defining episode was the transition of roles from attendants to nurses that provided a platform for the development of a professional identity (Nolan, 1993).

It wasn't until the mid twentieth century, when nursing theorists (mainly from the United States) developed theories and conceptualizations of the therapeutic relationship between nurses and clients (Barker, 1998). The development of the therapeutic relationship enabled mental health nurses to view patient care beyond the restricting boundaries of the medical model of care and to empathise with the patients being treated.

The therapeutic relationship is a concept held by many researchers to be fundamental to the identity of mental health nurses (Altshul, 1972, Barker, 1998, Peplau, 1952). Research into the understanding of the therapeutic relationship has given nursing an evidence base and introduced theories in the middle of the last century. Its origins can be traced to attendants' interpersonal practices in the asylum care in the 19th century. The dominance of the medical practitioners' perception of mental distress, and the working-class status of asylum attendants, prevented the development of professional opinion and understanding of the therapeutic relationship from a discipline predominantly involved in the care of inmates in the asylums. It was the influence of Hilegard Peplau (1952, 1962, 1963, 1987, 1990) and other nursing theorists (Altshul, 1972, Orlando, 1961, Render and Weiss, 1959, Travelbee, 1966) who described mental health nursing as a therapeutic relationship.

The meaning assigned to therapy or therapeutic has evolved throughout the years into specific meaning, but the constituents of the relationship between carer and cared for has become obscured by rhetoric and political correctness. It is accepted that the nature of therapy has changed and in particular become less physical since the custodial care of 19th century asylums (Chambers, 1998, O'Brien, 2001, Wilshaw, 1997). Asylum care was characterized by paternalistic, authoritarian regimes and as a care regime therapy was custodial and based on physical restraint (Weir, 1992).

BACKGROUND LITERATURE

The literature seems inclined to portray the therapeutic relationship as an elusive holy grail of psychiatric nursing endeavors. The contrary is actually the case, as the therapeutic relationship is the fundamental core and essence of the role of the psychiatric nurse (Altshul, 1972, Barker, 1998, Peplau 1952).

The literature indicates areas that require clarification from an evidence-based perspective and include attributes or attitudes, socialization process, skills, curative factors and how the connection between nurse and patient is enacted. These areas indicate the formation and intricacies within the relationship and how this process is defined as therapeutic. The literal definition of therapeutic is described as, contributing to the cure or soothing of a disease. Psychiatric nurses espouse practicing a therapeutic role and Peplau (1952), Altshul (1972), Forchuk and Brown (1989), Barker (1998) and Morrissey (2003) would maintain that the profession has embraced the role, but has not clearly identified in any sense the components of the relationship.

Scholars have quite clearly stated that the most appropriate approach to examine the therapeutic relationship is the interpretivist approach (Bevis, 1982, Chambers, 1998, Forchuk, 1991, Peavy, 1996). The theoretical process for examining the therapeutic relationship, which has emerged since the early work of Peplau (1952), emphasizes the understanding and interpretation of human experiences. The experiences elucidated in the literature focuses on personal factors, skills, curative factors and how the relationship is developed, but from the literature more questions are asked than answers elicited (Chambers 1998,

Sullivan 1998, Barker 1998). This study addresses these issues in an attempt to further the debate; the areas explored include how connection occurs in the therapeutic relationship, attitudes affecting the connection process, intuitive processes, curative factors and therapeutic skills used to develop the therapeutic relationship.

How Connection Occurs

Mental health care is delivered through a relationship between a clinician and a patient. Although this therapeutic relationship is of central importance for mental health care, it appears to be relatively neglected in psychiatric research. Empirical research has for the most part adopted concepts and methods developed in other disciplines such as psychotherapy and general medical practice.

Tickle-Dengen (2002) upon reviewing the available research suggested that communication functions within therapeutic relationships are fundamentally formulated in three concurrent and interlinked stages. These stages are the development of rapport, the development of a working alliance and maintenance of the working alliance. These stages appear to be formed similar to the map of counselling espoused by Burnard (1994), (Appendix 1).

Rowan (2002) describes three approaches to therapeutic liaisons, instrumental, authentic and transpersonal. The instrumental approach is universal as a way of being. It is learned responses or developmental material that is reinforced by socialization agents such as the family or mass media. The authentic approach requires some kind of initiation, which is quite readily acquired through therapy. It involves dealing with certain closed or subconscious aspects of existence, all those aspects of ourselves that we are initially reluctant to recognize. And the transpersonal approach also needs some kind of initiation, which has to be acquired through some of spiritual practice. It has to be some form of practice that teaches us, on an experiential level, that our boundaries are uncertain, that we do not live totally in isolation. It informs us that we are fundamentally divine, not limited by a narrow definition of our humanity.

Five types of therapeutic relationship were conceptualized by Clarkson (1994). These conceptualizations gave formal representation to the subjective experience of the therapeutic relationship within mental health nursing. The experiences are suggested to offer a theoretical framework to inform a working matrix fundamental to the relationship with patients.

The working alliance she describes as an agreement between carer and patient formulated to address a mutually agreed objective. The transferential or countertransferential relationship portrays a relationship during which essential issues described as dynamic that underpins the relationship itself and fundamentally forms the partnership. The developmentally needed relationship is described as initiating a corrective or informative function, during which identification of maladaptive interpersonal relationships are addressed. The I-Thou or person-to-person relationship is formed upon the subjective experience of the carer and the therapeutic essence is the product of the relationship itself, providing a forum for ventilation of experiences and emotions. The transpersonal relationship is described as factors extraneous to the relationship or spiritual elements of which quantification is limited and understanding in relation to what forms the relationship and how it operates is accepted as unknown or subconscious.

Psychiatric nursing is viewed by some to incorporate the role of developing therapeutic relationships (Gournay, 1996), whilst Forchuk (1991) views the therapeutic relationship as the essence and Peplau (1962) viewed it as the crux of psychiatric nursing practice. The relationship between psychiatric nurse and patient can be understood to be the development of self-awareness and healing for both parties (Peplau, 1952). A great deal is known about what psychiatric nurses are expected to do in forming therapeutic relationships, what is unsure is the meaning of this experience for the nurses. Most of the contemporary research on the therapeutic relationship has been conducted within a paradigm of positivist empirical research that emphasizes quantitative methods. While these investigations have provided vital information, they have been unable to capture the full intricacy of the factors of the relationship between nurse and patient. Therefore, the purpose of this research is to contribute to an increased knowledge of the meaning of the therapeutic relationship, from the perspective of psychiatric nurses.

Informed by the work of Peplau some scholars (Barker et al, 1995, Forchuk and Brown, 1989) have attempted to incorporate these conceptualizations into psychiatric nursing practice in the form of models and theories informing practice. Critics have argued that the ideologies and conceptualizations of the therapeutic relationship lack methodological objectivity and have encountered difficulty in measuring outcomes (Gournay, 1996).

Attitudes and Attributes

The successful formulation of the therapeutic relationship is dependent upon attitudes peculiar to the individual therapist. Attitudes adopted will depend to some extent on the particular therapist and his or her training in interpersonal skills. Rolfe (1990) argued that the theorist most carers associated with identification of attitudes is the theories of Rogers (1981). He identified three essential attitudes namely, genuineness, respect and empathy. However Omer (2000) would argue against this general conception stating that desirable attitudes in relation to the formulation, exploration and sustaining of therapeutic relationships have no universal correct application.

Empathy, warmth, and the therapeutic relationship have been shown to have more impact in relation to patients' perspective or therapeutic effect than more specialized or technical interventions (Lambert, 2001). Decades of research indicate that the provision of therapy is an interpersonal process in which a main curative component is the nature of the therapeutic relationship.

Personal attributes are individual within individual relationship and are transient between each relationship. Attributes most associated with the formation of a therapeutic relationship include global statements relating to effective relationship formation described by Rogers (1981) and Egan (1994). The person centered approach postulated by Rogers is primarily a way of being that finds expression in attitudes and behaviors that create a growth-promoting climate. It is a basic philosophy rather than simply a technique or a method. These attributes include genuineness, respect and empathy. However what isn't answered is whether all these factors need to be present and what degree practitioners are aware of the application within the therapeutic relationship.

Intuitive Processes

The research also shows that psychiatric nurses are at times practicing at an intuitive level; this begs the question; are psychiatric nurses practicing within his or her scope of practice? Conversely the therapeutic relationship is such an individualistic activity that some aspects of this relationship are described as immeasurable and need to remain such to allow spontaneity without measurement.

The influence of Peplau in relation to the issue of role identification and formalization of conscious practice cannot be understated; almost all commentators and researchers refer to Peplau as a significant catalyst for the examination of the role of the psychiatric nurse in relation to the therapeutic relationship (Barker, 1998, Chambers, 1998, Higgins et al, 1999, Melrose and Shapiro, 1999, Morrissey, 2003, O'Brien, 2001, Stickley, 2002, Sullivan, 1998, Whalley and Patton, 1999).

If the essence or crux of psychiatric nursing is the development of therapeutic relationships between psychiatric nurses and patients, research must clearly identify the components of such relationships. It is difficult to identify these components due to a number of factors involved, the two main factors being the convolution of variables involved and the assumptions relating to the location of therapeutic liaisons within the role of psychiatric nursing.

Altshul (1972) postulated the development of therapeutic relationships between nurse and patient was the result of intuition and not a consciously competent theory driven process. Therefore if the essence of psychiatric nursing is the development of therapeutic relationships and these interactions are as a result of intuition, ergo psychiatric nurses are neither utilizing evidence based practice nor are they performing their therapeutic role within the scope of professional practice.

LM. Weibe, (University of Toronto, Toronto, unpublished dissertation) described the therapeutic process as connection. Connection in this sense refers to the extent to, which a partnership evolves to address the therapeutic process. Connection occurs as a result of therapeutic techniques such as listening, questioning, clarifying, reflecting and interpreting. In addition to previously mentioned skills or techniques the extra therapeutic or extraneous factors, which appear to be undeterminable for example need further study. These extraneous factors are factors said to be based on intuition of individual psychiatric nurse practising mainly as a result of the socialization process.

Therapeutic Skills

Heron (1974) postulated a matrix when conducting his studies into humanistic existentialism, namely a six category intervention analysis. Heron cited interventions made by therapists to enable personal growth as existing within the following categories:

- Prescriptive- Making suggestions or recommending.
- Informative- Gives new knowledge or information to the patient.
- Confronting- Challenges restrictive or repetitive attitudes, beliefs or behaviours of the patient.
- Cathartic- Helps the patient to release tension through tears, trembling, angry sounds or laughter.
- Catalytic- Helps draw out information from or encourages self-discovery in the patient.

- Supportive- Affirms the worth of and is supportive of the patient.

Techniques or skills identified as being fundamental to formulating, sustaining and advancing the therapeutic relationship are generally accepted to fall into listening, questioning, encouraging ventilation, reflecting on content and clarifying (Minishull, 1982, Burnard, 1994).

Listening or active attending seems and is so easy; to listen carefully to what the patient is saying verbally and non-verbally and also to listen to what the therapist and patient is saying internally (Egan, 1994). Burnard, (1994) suggests that active listening means taking cognizance of metaphors, the descriptions, the value judgments and verbalizations of the counselor, as they are all indications of their personal world. Carkhuff, (1987) describes listening verbally and non-verbally as "attending" and this is the foundation of effective therapeutic relationships.

Any therapeutic intervention has to involve questions. Questioning has an important effect on therapeutic effectiveness, the number, type, intensity, open or closed and tone all have a bearing on the success or failure of the therapeutic relationship (Minishull, 1982). To some extent the skill of posing questions is allowing the individual to confront or challenge perspectives in their psyche. Researchers who agree that therapeutic relationships are helpful to the individual would concur that challenging or confronting the individuals' perceptions is a central component to the therapeutic nature of the relationship (Burnard 1991, Ellis and Dryden 1987).

The skill of encouragement is formed on the attitudes of the counselor, being hopeful and supportive and conveying this attitude to the person. Encouragement is more than just a verbal exchange or a "pat on the back" (Tschudin, 1995). Encouraging a person to talk about their inner most fears, secrets, problems or anxieties, involves a range of attitudes including empathy, warmth, genuineness or transparency and as stated by Rogers (1981) unconditional positive regard.

The ability to attend and encourage ventilation in tandem with an ability to explore the verbalizations by echoing statements made during the conversation to encourage the extrapolation of issues is vital to continue the relationship. The issues themselves require a complete and clear understanding. Often a partial understanding of issues provokes anxiety for the patient and merely talking through them with a second party clarifies the issues for the person, without any intervention from the therapist (Nelson-Jones, 1993).

Curative Factors

The notion of therapy implies some form of development or positive change in the individual. The notion of how individuals change is described by some commentators as curative (AC. Berkery, Adelphi University, NY, unpublished dissertation, Stickley, 2002), alternatively some scholars dispute the notion of a cure and would maintain the role of the psychiatric nurse is to optimize and maintain good health (Barker, 1998, Gournay, 1996).

To formulate a rationale to approach the understanding of the therapeutic relationship is partly located in research undertaken in the field previously. One such study identified seven elements related to change producing elements:

- The formulation of a relationship determined by real and fantasised qualities of carer and patient.
- The expression of emotional tension.
- Learning or development of understanding.
- Operant conditioning based on approval or disapproval and corrective responses during the therapeutic experience.
- Suggestion and persuasion, overt and covert.
- Development of self-awareness.
- Repeated reality testing and reflection.
- (Marmor, 1982)

The fundamental principles described are all important elements of the therapeutic process within relationships. The formation of the relationship has been described as a journey with expectancy, outcomes and co-operation. The journey is in partnership and AC. Berkery, (Adelphi University, NY, unpublished dissertation) descriptively postulated a double helix to describe both therapist and patient traveling this journey together. What isn't described and is significant to psychiatric nursing practice are the components formulating this journey to ensure conscious competence in nursing practice. It isn't questionable whether the therapeutic relationship is the essence (Peplau, 1952) or forms part of the role, what is imperative is that psychiatric nurses are aware of the significance of the therapeutic relationship within his or her role as mental health practitioners.

The curative elements described relate to how the psychiatric nurse engages with the patient and what elements of this engagement are curative or therapeutic. The curative elements can be described as engagement factors and developmental factors.

KEY STUDIES

Having reviewed the literature in relation to the therapeutic relationship and related areas of interpersonal relations and communication in psychiatric nursing a few relevant studies were discovered. These studies were determined to be of significance to this investigation due to the similarities of their aims and methodologies. The purpose of this study is to examine in detail psychiatric nurses perceptions of what constitutes the therapeutic relationship. The following section therefore reviews these studies in more detail.

Stickley (2002) although writing about counseling in mental health nursing describes one of the objectives of the study to explore mental health nurses experiences of the therapeutic relationship. The study research design was a grounded theory design involving five unstructured interviews of mental health nurses. The selection of nurses was psychiatric nurses qualified for less than two years, which would appear to this author insufficient time to gain exposure to the phenomena under investigation. What the study does describe is the role of the psychiatric nurse and discovers that psychiatric nurses are in a profession that is demanding and insufficiently trained to perform that role. This is significant to this investigation as one of the questions raised relates to the degree psychiatric nurses develop therapeutic relationships consciously and competently. The findings of the study produced four major themes:

- Mental Health Nursing is a stressful job.
- Nurse training did not equip them for one-to-one counseling.
- Effective supervision would assist counseling in psychiatric nursing.
- More effective training would benefit the nurse in this aspect of their work.

One unfortunate observation in relation to the study is the answers gleaned are more encompassing than the questions asked. The study makes a claim that changes in training methods are warranted, but these changes relate to counseling skills training. This is an aspect of psychiatric nurse training but the study does not apply this to how a psychiatric nurse utilizes counseling in his or her practice. The study makes a claim that it illuminates a patient perspective and identifies what patient requirements may be. The study in general seemed far too broad ranging and as such appeared not to investigate in any detail any aspect proposed to be investigated.

LM. Weibe (University of Toronto, Toronto, unpublished dissertation) studied the therapeutic relationship's essential yet elusive nature by exploring clients' and therapists' experiences of connection in the therapeutic relationship. Twelve participants were drawn from a Depression Project. Consistent with a two-person model of relationship, both clients and therapists in six therapeutic relationships were interviewed about their experiences of connection in actual videotaped therapy sessions. Interpersonal process recall (IPR) interviews were conducted in order to capture the here and now, subjective meaning and experience of connection for the participants. A grounded theory analysis was utilized in order to integrate both the clients' and the therapists' subjective experiences of connection. The resultant theory determined that connection in the therapeutic relationship is the experience of sharing a subjective world. The here and now experience of connection ranges from the ordinary to the profound, and it is grounded in the relationship in which it exists. Therefore, the experience of connection in the therapeutic relationship is unique. For both participants in the relationship, sharing a subjective world in the therapeutic relationship is coming to know, and interact with, the client's inner world. The mutual work of therapy is connecting, as is the interactive process of building the therapeutic relationship. The culmination of these choices is the experience, for both client and therapist, of connecting with the client's subjective world. For the therapist, this is the experience of meeting and sharing another's inner world. For the client, this is the experience of knowing his/her own inner world. Therefore, in connecting with another, one ultimately connects with oneself. This is the significance of connection in the therapeutic relationship.

The study although rigorous and describing vividly the nature of how patient and nurse engage in the therapeutic relationship, what it does not do is to posit a theory as described by Glaser and Strauss (1967) or Strauss and Corbin (1990). It is as described by Priest et al (2002) analytic description. Methodologically the study is open to criticism due to the selection of participants and the conditions of data collection. Videotaping of the interviews under real life situations is difficult, if not impossible due to the Hawthorne effect. This relates to how the participant who is knowingly being studied alters his or her behavior to produce a more favorable view of them in the study. The question is posed therefore how authentic is the data collected due to the fact the participants may have altered his or her natural behavior due the awareness they are being studied.

AC. Berkery (Adelphi University, NY, unpublished dissertation) studied nurse psychotherapists' experiences of the meaning of the therapeutic relationship. Ontological hermeneutics was the mode of inquiry used to explore the meaning of this human experience. An interpretation of the meaning of being in a therapeutic relationship was derived from in-depth unstructured interviews with five experienced nurse psychotherapists. The interpretation of meaning was achieved through a process of continuous dialogue and reflection with the text. The interpretation revealed shared practices and common meanings among the therapists. Two constitutive patterns and seven themes emerged. The first constitutive pattern "In the Trenches or Lost in Stories" and the three themes that constitute it, describes the ways the therapists travelled with their clients on the journey of psychotherapy. The second constitutive pattern, "The Begging Bowl: Allowing an Opening for Possibilities" describes the how of the therapeutic relationship and consists of four themes. The therapeutic relationship is described as a journey, and pictured as moving in the shape of a double helix. The therapist and client travel side-by-side bound together by the bonds of the therapeutic relationship. It is clear that the therapists were not distant objective observers in the relationship; they were intimately and actively committed to their clients and their journey together. The relationship is not one way; the relationship is healing for the therapists as well and they grow in their ability to provide care authentically. The intent of this interpretive research was not to gather facts, but rather, to initiate a dialogue about experiences with therapeutic relationships in the practice of nurse psychotherapists. This research raised many questions that can only be addressed by continuing dialogue among nurse clinicians, educators and researchers.

KJ. Evans (University Microfilms International, Auburn University, AL, unpublished dissertation) study was to investigate patient and therapist perceptions of the therapeutic relationship and to develop a theory about the relationship based on these findings. An existing model of the therapeutic relationship was explicated and used as point of comparison to the findings of this study. A book co-written by therapist Irvin Yalom and his patient was used as the data source for this analysis. This book contained narratives written by both therapist and patient after each therapy session over the course of their twenty-month therapy. These narratives contained patient and therapist perceptions of their experiences in therapy. The text of these narratives was analysed qualitatively based on established procedures of grounded theory analysis. This method yielded 482 meaning units, which were thought to depict central relationship themes over the course of therapy. A hierarchical categorization structure was developed from these meaning units, in which categories were established to explain relationships among items and to illuminate core themes that emerged from the data set. The three categories of "Third-Party Participants in the Relationship," "Patient Participation in the Relationship," and "Therapist Participation in the Relationship" formed the core categories within which all other categories were grouped. Based on the findings, a theory of the therapeutic relationship was developed that sought to explain the possible dynamics from which the categorization scheme emerged. A comparison was made between an established theory of the relationship and the findings yielded by this study.

This study claims to be a grounded theory method, although the methods of analysis were utilised, the philosophical assumptions informing grounded theory were lacking. This can be illustrated by the method of data collection and analysis; complete emersion in the data is advocated in grounded theory (Glaser, 1992), however half the data is collected through a hermeneutic analysis of a previous therapeutic relationship by Irvin Yalom. Grounded theory is also informed by human interaction and analysis of symbols this study is an analysis of text and therefore methodologically questionable.

Gaps in the Literature

The review of the literature indicates that the therapeutic relationship, although the essence of psychiatric nursing (Peplau, 1952) is not understood to any great extent. Attempts have been made to empirically locate aspects of the therapeutic relationship in nursing epistemology (AC. Berkery, Adelphi University, NY, unpublished dissertation, KJ. Evans, University Microfilm International, Auburn University, AL, unpublished dissertation, Stickley, 2002, LM. Weibe, University of Toronto, Toronto, unpublished dissertation). On the whole comment on how psychiatric nurses perceive their role in relation to developing therapeutic relationships has been as result of the location of psychiatric nursing within the American neo-Freudian tradition by Peplau (1952). This study offers the opportunity to provide empirical evidence to explore the phenomena in Irish psychiatric nursing, hither to unexplored.

A common theme identified in a great deal of the literature relating to the therapeutic relationship is that psychiatric nurses are practicing at an intuitive level (Altshul, 1972, Barker, 1998, Morrissey, 2003, LM. Weibe, University of Toronto, Toronto, unpublished dissertation). This intuitive development of the therapeutic relationship is not merely the use of personal experience; it is an application of developmentally acquired knowledge relating to human experience and the addition of acquired knowledge relating to interpersonal skills. The degree of understanding attributed to the constituents of the therapeutic relationship is minimal (Barker,1998, Gournay, 1996, Stickley, 2002). Perhaps the reason for this is; to fully understand and to adjust practice in the light of research findings would fundamentally challenge psychiatric nursing practice, which is seen as a profession based on common sense and intuitive practice (Altshul, 1972).

As provided by the evidence in the literature interpersonal relationships and the therapeutic process within psychiatric nursing relationships has been the subject of discourse for approximately three decades. It is not coincidental that Peplau postulated her ideas at this time however consensus of opinion suggests that components formulating the therapeutic relationship have not been fully extrapolated (Barker, 1998, Forchuk, 1991, Stickley, 2002).

What is clearly stated is the most appropriate research methodology is located within the interpretivist paradigm (Altshul, 1972, Barker, 1998, Peplau, 1990). If psychiatric nurses consider the positivist perspective appropriate to explore human experiences and relationships. This may be a reflection of professional insecurity and as cited by Bevis (1982). Nurses should be confident to utilize appropriate, but less favorable approaches to research to advance knowledge and nursing science. The purpose of this study is to explore psychiatric nurses' perceptions of the constituents of the therapeutic relationship and the evidence supplied by the literature would indicate possibly the most appropriate method would be a grounded theory approach as the therapeutic relationship is a circumstance driven process. One of the aims of grounded theory research as described by Strauss and Corbin (1990) is to guide practitioners' practice and to develop a basic knowledge. What the literature is also generating is a need to advance an epistemological basis for the exploration of professional practice and relate this issue to the impact on the clarification of the role of the psychiatric nurse.

Findings of key studies indicated that it is important when developing therapeutic relationships that the various players in the relationship are aware of who does what, why and how (KJ. Evans, University Microfilms International, Auburn University, AL, unpublished dissertation). What was also clearly identified in the key studies was that this is a partnership between psychiatric nurse and the patient and this partnership is a journey into the world of the patient (AC. Berkery, Adelphi University, NY, unpublished dissertation). LM. Weibe (University of Toronto, Toronto, unpublished dissertation) describes vividly the nature of how connection occurs between patient and nurse and describes this relationship as an equal partnership. What is described illuminates the debate surrounding the nature of the therapeutic relationship, what it does not do is concretely dissect and explain the components of the therapeutic relationship that is the objective of this study. Appendix 2 indicates how the literature review has significance in this study to enable the sensitising of concepts and to highlight gaps in the literature.

Chapter two, which follows, explains the theoretical perspective, method and methodology of the study. A detailed description of how a grounded theory investigation is appropriate to study the stated phenomena is discussed.

REFERENCES

Altshul A. (1972) A Study of interaction patterns in acute psychiatric wards. Edinburgh, Churchill Livingstone.

Barker P. (1998) The future of the theory of interpersonal relation? A personal reflection on Peplau's legacy. *Journal of Psychiatric and Mental Health Nursing.* 5, 213-220.

Barker P., Reynolds B. and Ward T. (1995) The proper focus of nursing: a critique of the 'caring' ideology. *International Journal of Nursing Studies.* 32, 386-397.

Bevis EO. (1982) Curriculum building in nursing- a process, 3rd edn. St Louis, CV Mosby.

Burnard P. (1991) Acquiring minimum counselling skills. NursingStandard 5(46):37-39.

Burnard P. (1994) Counselling Skills for Health Professionals. (2nd Ed). London, Chapman and Hall.

Carkhuff RR. (1987) The Art of helping, 6th edn. Amherst, Human Resource Development Press.

Chambers M. (1998) Interpersonal mental health nursing: Research issues and challenges. *Journal of Psychiatric and Mental Health Nursing.* 5, 203-211.

Clarkson P. (1994) The psychotherapeutic relationship. In: The Handbook of Psychotherapy, (eds Clarkson P. and Pokorny M.), pp 28-48. London, Routledge.

Egan G. (1994) The skilled helper, 5th edn. Pacific grove, California, Brooks/Cole.

Ellis A. and Dryden W. (1987) The Practice of Rational Emotive Therapy. New York, Springer.

Forchuk C. (1991) A comparison of the works of Peplau and Orlando. *Archives of Psychiatric Nursing.* V, 38-45.

Forchuk C. and Brown B. (1989) Establishing a nurse-client relationship. *Journal of Psychosocial Nursing and Mental Health Services.* 27, 30-34.

Glaser BG. (1992) Basics of grounded theory analysis: emergence vs forcing. Mill Valley, California, Sociology Press.

Glaser BG. and Strauss A. (1967) The discovery of grounded theory: strategies for qualitative research. New York, Aldine de Gruyter.

Gournay K. (1996) Schizophrenia: a review of the contemporary literature and implications for mental health nursing theory practice and education. *Journal of Psychiatric and Mental Health Nursing.* 4, 441-446.

Heron J. (1974) The peer learning community. Guildford, University of Surrey.

Higgins R., Hurst K. and Wistow G. (1999) Nursing acute patients: A quantitative and qualitative study. *Journal of Advanced Nursing.* 29(1), 52-63.

Hutchinson SA. and Wilson HS. (2001) Grounded theory: the method, In: Nursing research: A qualitative perspective, 3rd edn. (ed Munhall PL). pp 209-243. London, Jones and Bartlett.

Lambert MJ. (2001) Research summary on the therapeutic relationship and psychotherapy outcome. Psychotherapy: Theory, Research, Practice, Training. 38(4), 357-361.

Marmor J. (1982) Change in psychoanylitic treatment. In: Curative Factors in Dynamic Psychotherapy, (ed Slipp S), pp 60-70. New York, Magraw Hill.

Melrose S. and Shapiro B. (1999) Student's perceptions of their psychiatric mental health clinical nursing experience: a personal construct theory exploration. *Journal of Advanced Nursing.* 30(6), 1451-1458.

Minishull D. (1982) Counselling in psychiatric nursing Part 1.*Nursing Times.* 78, 1201-1202.

Morrissey MV. (2003) Becoming a mental health nurse: a qualitative study (part 1). The International Journal of Psychiatric Nursing Research. 8(3), 963-971.

Nelson-Jones R. (1993) Practical counselling and helping skills, How to use the lifeskills helping model, 3rd edn. New York, Cassell.

Nolan PW. (1993) A history of the training of asylum nurses. *Journal of Advanced Nursing.* 18, 1193-1201.

O'Brien AJ. (2001) The therapeutic relationship: historical development and contemporary significance. *Journal of Psychiatric and Mental Health Nursing.* 8, 129-137.

Omer H. (2000) Troubles in the therapeutic relationship: A pluralistic perspective. *Journal of Clinical Psychology.* 56(2), 201-210.

Orlando IJ. (1961) The dynamic nurse-patient relationship. New York, G.P. Putnam's Sons.

Peavy RV. (1996) Counselling as a culture of healing. *British Journal of Guidance Counselling.* 24(1), 141-150.

Peplau HE. (1952) Interpersonal relations in nursing. New York, Putnam.

Peplau HE. (1962) Interpersonal techniques: The crux of psychiatric nursing. *American Journal of Nursing.* 62, 50-54.

Peplau HE. (1963) The heart of nursing: interpersonal relations. *The Canadian Nurse.* 61,273-275.

Peplau HE. (1987) Interpersonal constructs for nursing practice. *Nurse Education Today.* 7, 201-208.

Peplau HE. (1990) Interpersonal relations model: Principles and general applications. In: Psychiatric and Mental Health Nursing: Theory and Practice. (eds Reynolds W. and Cormack D.), pp 87-132. London, Chapman and Hall.

Priest H., Roberts P. and Woods L. (2002) An overview of three different approaches to the interpretation of qualitative data. Part 1: theoretical issues. Nurse Researcher. 10, 1, 30-42.

Render HW. and Weiss MO. (1959) Nurse-Patient relationships in psychiatry, 2nd edn. New York, McGraw-Hill.

Rogers C. (1981) Client-centred Therapy. London, Constable.

Rolfe G. (1990) The assessment of therapeutic attitudes in the psychiatric setting. *Journal of Advanced Nursing.* 15, 564-570.

Rowan J. (2002) The three approaches to a therapeutic relationship: Instrumental, authentic, transpersonal. Counselling Psychology Review. 17(4), 3-10.

Stickley T. (2002) Counselling and mental health nursing: a qualitative study. *Journal of Psychiatric and Mental Health Nursing.* 9, 301-308.

Strauss A. and Corbin J. (1990) Basics of qualitative research. Newbury Park CA, Sage.

Sullivan P. (1998) Therapeutic interaction and mental health nursing. Nursing Standard. 12, 45, 39-42.

Tickle-Dengen L. (2002) Client-centered practice, therapeutic relationship, and the use of research evidence. *American Journal of Occupational Therapy.* 56(4), 470-474.

Travelbee J. (1966) Interpersonal aspects of nursing. Philadelphia, F.A. Davis Company.

Tschudin V. (1995) Counselling skills for nurses, 2nd Edn. London, Baliere Tindall.

Whalley J. and Patton H. (1999) 'Freedom of speech': promoting the use of counselling skills. Mental Health Nursing. 19(1), 20-23.

Weir RJ. (1992) An experimental course of lectures on moral treatment for mentally ill people. *Journal of Advanced Nursing.* 17, 390-395.

Wilshaw G. (1997) Integration of therapeutic approaches: a new direction for mental health nurses? *Journal of Advanced Nursing.* 26, 15-19.

Chapter Two

THE STUDY DESIGN

This chapter begins with the methods and methodology used to explore psychiatric nurses perceptions of the constituents of the therapeutic relationship. The first section of the chapter begins with a discussion of the naturalistic paradigm in relation to social science research. This is discussed in relation to nursing epistemology. The discussion informs the rationale for the choice of methods for this investigation. Grounded theory design is explained in detail and relates the method to the research question. The sampling processes are examined and the negotiation of access procedures explained. The process of data collection and data analysis are described in detail. Ethical considerations are discussed in relation to the study.

NATURALISTIC PARADIGM IN RESEARCH

Identifying the approaches informing research methods is crucial to maintain authenticity, rigour and appropriateness. Ontology refers to assumptions made in relation to what constitutes reality (Guba and Lincoln, 1994). Reality in naturalistic inquiry is referred to in relation to this study when choosing a research approach. It identifies whether reality is external to the individual or a result of the persons' consciousness.

Epistemology refers to the way in which the knowledge of reality is constructed, it considers how and what is knowledge and describes the relationship between researcher and what may be known (Blaikie, 1993).

Research in psychiatric nursing and nursing in general is predominantly within the field of social sciences. Social science research exists within two research paradigms. These research paradigms differ fundamentally in relation to the most effective means of generating knowledge.

The positivist paradigm considers there to be an objective truth that is independent from the subject. Positivist research is linear, analytical, deductive and tests hypotheses. Research within this paradigm is concerned with the measurement of observable data and manipulation of the data to discover universal laws (Paley, 2000).

The naturalistic paradigm considers there is no single objective reality and that reality is constructed by the interpretation of each individual, including the researcher (Schumacher and Gortner, 1992). The presenting phenomena are studied in their own context and are specific to circumstance. Naturalistic inquiry seeks to gain knowledge through understanding how individuals interpret their own circumstances (Treacy and Hyde, 1999). To this end data are collected by interviewing and observing participants in situ. The three main naturalistic methods of research are ethnography, phenomenology and grounded theory.

Grounded theory is informed by the constructionist research paradigm, that emphasizes social reality is produced and reproduced by social actors (Norton, 1999). As a result the constructionist perspective maintains there are many constructions of reality. The constructionist research paradigm understands researchers are inseparable from formation of social realities; due to the fact researchers construct the worlds they research. In constructionist research ontology and epistemology merge due to the knower being inseparable from whatever can be known within the overall construction of a particular reality (Annells, 1996).

Within the constructionist paradigm individuals are perceived not to encounter phenomena and identify meaning singularly. Humans moreover are introduced to a world of meaning and enter a social sphere and describe an environment of significant symbols. In relation to the proposed study, psychiatric nurses enter the field of psychiatric nursing and are socialised into particular practice and the culture reveals meaning in relation to reality. Ergo, constructionists view all meaningful reality is socially constructed and to identify meaning would necessitate epistemology to be within the culture of psychiatric nursing and constructed from interactions between actors (Crotty, 1998).

In this sense what is maintained to be reality is the meaning attributed to social interactions in the context of culturally adapted phenomena. Constructionists suppose that society is actively and creatively encountered and emphasised by individual players within social settings.

The three notions of ontology, epistemology and methodology are reciprocally related in that ontology defines epistemology and methodology is informed by both ontology and epistemology. Grounded theory is located in the interpretivist approach of constructionism, which informs the theoretical framework of symbolic interactionism.

Naturalistic inquiry is the most appropriate approach to use in this study. The research question is what determines the method of research adopted and in this case the research question seeks to ascertain what psychiatric nurses perceive to be the constituents of the therapeutic relationship. Naturalistic inquiry accepts that there are many perceptions of what constitutes reality and the objective of this study is to explore the perceptions of psychiatric nurses' as to what forms the relationship between nurse and patient and what makes this relationship therapeutic.

CHOOSING A RESEARCH APPROACH

The objective of this research is to develop a theory to inform conscious psychiatric nursing practice in relation to forming therapeutic relationships. To date research described as grounded theory has been largely descriptive. As stated by Glaser (1992) and Priest et al (2002) research described as grounded theory utilising well-known analytical methods falls short of the formation of theories and is merely analytical description.

Strauss and Corbin (1990) describe one of the purposes of research is to guide practitioners' practices and to develop a basic knowledge. In this study the objective is to form a theory relating to constituents of the therapeutic relationship to inform professional psychiatric nursing practice. Building theory implies interpreting data that must be conceptualised and the concepts related to a view of reality. This view of reality is formed upon results of data analysis that provides a framework to develop a theory. The process of analysis leading to the postulation of a theory is a systematic approach to build on existing knowledge and to integrate a priori knowledge with new knowledge.

A grounded theory study is derived inductively by studying the phenomenon produced in the study area. Significantly the two founder fathers of grounded theory Barney Glaser and Anselm Strauss differed in relation to analysis of data Glaser (1992) maintaining that emergence relied purely upon the participants' views of reality. However Strauss and Corbin (1990) posited that to formulate a theory with any meaning it must be formed through evidence from literature, professional experience and personal experience and to some extent 'force' the formulation of a theory. The following section identifies the theoretical background informing grounded theory.

Theoretical Perspective Informing Grounded Theory Research

Social psychologists Mead (1934) and Blumer (1969) postulated theories relating to human interaction, defining social interaction in terms of symbols or language. Symbolic Interactionism holds three basic assumptions:

- Human beings act toward things on the basis of the meaning that things have for them.
- The meaning of things in life rises out of the social interaction that a person has with others.
- Meanings are modified through an interpretive process in which people engage when they deal with things that they encounter.

(Blumer, 1969) Benzies and Allen (2001) maintain that symbolic interactionism is also influenced by Darwin's theory of evolution, citing that the environment is dynamic and human behaviour is determined by adapting to the environment. Symbolic interactionism extracts from this theory that the individual and the environment have a dependant relationship through formation of relationships.

This philosophy underpins the symbolic interactionist perspective, proponents of which argue that the socialisation process is not just about individuals learning about their society but is also a process whereby they develop the ability to think and to absorb information and shape it according to their needs (Ritzer, 1996). In this way, social life is defined by the meanings that we attach to objects. For symbolic interactionists the role of language is of central importance as they regard language as an enormous set of symbols.

Because of human beings ability to understand symbols, people can adjust the behaviour they will employ as, amongst other things, they are aware of the potential consequences of any action, or can learn what the consequences are likely to be. Erving Goffman, who famously interpreted social action as a dramatic performance, further developed this understanding of human behaviour, as a series of symbolic interactions (Goffman, 1961).

The objective of this study is to explore psychiatric nurses' perceptions of the constituents of the therapeutic relationship, the method chosen answers this question as the perceptions of their reality is the research objective. The methodology chosen, namely grounded theory allowed a systematic, dense, explanatory theory to be developed (Preist et al, 2002).

SAMPLE

This section of the study seeks to identify a rationale for the chosen sample. The section will explore how access to the participants was obtained. The section will also identify a rationale for including certain participants and not including others and provide clear criteria for making these decisions. The section will review how the sample was selected and review the process to achieve this selection.

Negotiating Access

The research was conducted in an Irish psychiatric hospital setting; the identified participants were sufficiently exposed to the research phenomenon. Access to conduct the research was negotiated with a number of gatekeepers before the commencement of the study. These gatekeepers included the Director of Psychiatric Nursing Services, the Programme Manager, Ward Managers and the Individual nurses involved in the study. The researcher must seek to gain ethical approval to conduct the study from appropriate authorities. Formal ethical approval was sought and granted by the Director of Nursing (appendix 5, appendix 8). Formal approval to conduct the study is paramount to good practice in research, protecting the researcher and the participant (Mason, 1996).

Inclusion Criteria

The sample nurses were generic psychiatric nurses with no post registration training in counseling or related courses that could bias the data towards a counseling orientation. The research refers to psychiatric nurses' perceptions of the constituents of the therapeutic relationship that could be biased by extra training in counseling. The size of the sample was determined by saturation of theoretical codes (Strauss and Corbin, 1990). Saturation occurs if the researcher can use the data to answer questions in relation to cause, context and consequences of a code. In this study it was assumed that saturation would occur with a sample of six participants. Saturation was not achieved in this particular study due to the small sample size and the limited amount of time to reach a conclusion to the study. In relation to time constraints, the sample size of six balances saturation and expediency. To locate a purposive sample, the inclusion criteria in this study required:

- Voluntary participation.
- Registered on the psychiatric division of nurses.
- Nurses who have been registered longer than two years and no longer than ten years.
- Nurses who have no additional training in counseling or related field.

The sample of psychiatric nurses was post registration nurses of between two and ten years. The assumption was that nurses trained over two years would have sufficient exposure to form an educated opinion. The ten-year threshold is identified due to; nurses trained beyond this period would have been educated in a different curriculum.

Sample Selection

Having located the research question and identified research methods it is incumbent upon the researcher to define and access a sample. The sample for this study was a purposive sample of six psychiatric nurses. The rationale for Purposive sampling as opposed to any other form of sampling lies with the selected methodology. Grounded theory requires information to be obtained from a particular research population this population must hold the information required. In this study the information required is located in psychiatric nurses who are post qualification between two and ten years, this would ensure sufficient exposure to the phenomenon of the therapeutic relationship, without crossing educational differences. The Assistant Director of nursing department was requested to furnish me with a list of names of nurses who fulfil the inclusion criteria. Nurses who met the inclusion criteria were selected from the list. The nurses who were selected to participate were requested to on the basis of the research question and the notion that they hold the required answers to this research question.

Sample Selection Process

Upon receiving the list of nurses who fulfill the selection inclusion criteria I began to invite individuals to participate in the study. In this study the target population was a purposive and volunteer sample. The participants' involvement in the study was qualified by an explanation of the research question and their role in the study. The initial contact was made with each participant by telephone. One identified nurse decided not to participate in the study due to prior commitments and one other prospective participant could not find the time to participate in the study.

Following the initial contact I arranged interviews on an individual basis and arranged to meet each participant half an hour before each interview. This initial interview was to informally clarify objectives of the study, inform participants of their rights of participation and to gain informed consent. The negotiation of access was required to be explicit in relation to study objectives. Approval or informed consent was required from the authorities and from the participants. This study identified a clear agenda and the ethical approval for the study was made explicit (Appendix 5). Informed consent was sought from each participant, disseminating explicit information in relation to future use of the material, researcher's right to publish the results of the study and the participants' right to withdraw consent (Maykut and Morehouse, 1994). Each participant was asked to read an informed consent form and sign to express approval and understanding of their rights (Appendix 4).

As consistent with a grounded theory method of research, theoretical sampling or purposive sampling was adopted. This process involves deciding on the sample size and type prior and during the research. This purposive sample is based on the type of questions requiring to be answered by participants and information required to be collected to answer the question. Appendix two indicates that the process of grounded theory requires clear purposive sampling or theoretical sampling as in this study.

Data Collection

The framework of data collection was semi-structured depth interviews; the topic guide will include themes identified by the background literature. Appendix 3 identifies themes in relation to the research question elicited from the literature. The interviews were transcribed and analyzed as identified by Strauss and Corbin, (1990). A pilot of the proposed interviews was undertaken prior to the study to unsure the interview is focused, fits the study, is timed well and is conducted under the exact arrangements as the actual interviews.

Access to the tapes and transcripts were strictly limited to the researcher and relevant academic staff supervising the researcher. The study has been reported in the first person as the researcher is co-participant in the research process. The interviews were six interviews of fifty to sixty minutes duration, to best enable saturation of data, whilst cognizant of expediency and time constraints.

Saturation refers to completeness of theoretical information and no new concepts are emerging. New descriptive data may be added but without altering codes the data will be exhausted and repetitive. The researcher by repeating questions of emerging data eventually acquires a sense of closure.

The Interview Guide (Appendix 3)

An interview guide was developed informed by the available literature and upon my own experiences as a psychiatric nurse. It comprised open questions and was used as a reference to prompt me during the interviews, as I am a novice researcher. It was sufficiently structured to allow me to deviate from the guide to explore the participants' world and to expand on important information that was emerging. The guide was amended regularly, following information gained from previous interviews, but the main tenants of the guide remained constant.

A GANT chart (appendix 6) outlines the sequence of events through the research process. Resources identified for the study are detailed in appendix 7 and include technical and manpower issues.

Pilot Study

Pilot studies are small representations of the proposed investigation. They are performed in an attempt to determine any problems in the research design in relation to data collection procedures. By undertaking a pilot of the proposed study the researcher can make modifications to the data collection process, informed by the lessons from the pilot exercise (Polit and Hungler, 1995). In this investigation the objective of the pilot study was to test the interview schedule and to ascertain whether the answers given and the data collected were appropriate to answer the research question. In addition to testing structural and logistical requirements the pilot study aimed to allow the researchers to practice interactive skills such as listening skills, asking questions and interpersonal skills (Keats, 2000).

The pilot interview was a useful exercise in this particular study, to identify repetitions in the original interview guide that where altered in subsequent interviews. I also learned that the timing of the interview was good and gave sufficient scope to explore areas as they emerged from the participants. I changed one particular question that was attempting to explore perceived attitudes of the patient towards developing therapeutic relationships. This question in hindsight was inappropriate and difficult for the nurse to answer. Subsequent studies examining the therapeutic relationship from the perspective of the patient may address this anomaly.

The Interviews

Individual semi-structured interviews were chosen as a method of data collection. This method enabled a flexible approach to data collection and fits with grounded theory methodology (Morse and Field, 1985). More structured data collection methods would not be consistent with a grounded theory approach, as it would not allow the participants the opportunity to expand on their responses to the questions posed in the interview. Prior to the interview commencing I sought permission to record the interview and to take notes as required, each participant granted this. I reassured each participant of the commitment to maintain confidentiality and anonymity prior to each interview. Six depth interviews were conducted.

PROCEDURAL ISSUES

Arranging interviews seems and sounds an easy process, however in practice a great deal needs to be considered. The process initially involved searching the staff records system for the purposive sample as specified. The names of nurses identified in the search had to be liaised with to arrange appropriate times and venues. Extraneous variables such as identified in one particular case had to be considered. This particular nurse was on night duty at the time and I had to consider would the fact they were on night duty impact on the results of the study. I needed to consider would an interview at night although convenient and expedient, would it be different in any way to the remainder of interviews conducted during the day. My conclusion was to allow the individual to complete their night duty and conduct all the interviews under similar conditions.

The interviews generally went well and following the pilot interview the question were amended slightly in the light of the data emerging. The data and the nature of the findings produced in the pilot interview were sufficient to be included in the general data collection. The interviews were conducted in the participants' place of work, in a quiet area, undisturbed. Each participant volunteered and co-operated with the ethos of the study and provided a substantial amount of significant data. The following chapter is an analysis of the emerging data.

The interviews generally went well and the interview guide (appendix three) assisted in keeping me focussed. My confidence increased as I became more confident and familiar with the interview guide and the emerging information. Each successive interview added to information from the previous interview and I began to synthesise the emerging issues to the previous issues. Prior to each interview the equipment was checked including, spare batteries and the microphone was functioning. The interviews took place in the participants' place of work. The reason for this was to ensure that most interviews were consistent and that the individuals involved were comfortable in the environment. In addition, if granted permission for an hour away from the work place the participants may be encouraged to engage more fully.

The transcribing of the interviews was very much underestimated; it was very tedious and time consuming. The interviews on average lasted between fifty minutes and one hour, these interviews took approximately nine to eleven hours to transcribe onto a text document. The interviews were hand written from listening to the tape over and rewinding. These notes written by hand were then transcribed to a text document and adjusted appropriately. The quality of the tape recordings was sufficient to enable me to easily transfer the data from verbal to written material. This was significant as it meant no data was lost.

Following the interviews the data was transcribed and analysed. This analysis is discussed in the following section. Interviewees or participants can be identified in the findings by reference to participant and the page of the transcript, for example p1.2.

Data Analysis

Analysis of the data was according to methods described by Strauss and Corbin (1990); namely grounded theory. This is a constant comparative method, best described as a cyclical process involving inductive and deductive processes. The following section describes how the data were dealt with upon being collected, the analysis process to the formulation of a theory. The objective of this research is to provide a theory in relation to psychiatric nurses' perceptions of the constituents of the therapeutic relationship.

Handling the Data

When the interviews were transcribed any names reference to names or places was erased or references were coded to maintain anonymity. When the data was transcribed the tapes were played simultaneously to readings the transcripts to verify the content as correct. These transcripts were copied and stored in a locked draw; the original documents were used for analysis. When the interviews were typed there was a total of thirty nine thousand eight hundred and three words in the six interview transcripts. This wordage amounted to fifty four pages of text only format in courier font.

Analyzing the Data

Grounded theory method states that the development of theory should be as a result of analysis of data and not prior knowledge (Glaser, 1992, Glaser and Strauss, 1967). This process should be a clear consistent process that reveals the analytical process. In grounded theory two positions have been adopted by the two founders, namely Anselm Strauss and Barney Glaser. Glaser (1992) maintains the development of theory should be grounded in the data and the theory should emerge.

Strauss and Corbin (1990) posited that the method should not merely be descriptive, but should explain phenomena elicited from the data (Stern, 1994). This fundamental difference explains the rationale for adopting either a 'Glaserian' or 'Strausserian' approach. Having conducted a review of literature and the notion that a priori knowledge will influence the 'forcing' of a theory to explain psychiatric nurses' perceptions of the constituents of the therapeutic relationship, Strauss and Corbin's (1990) explanation of grounded theory best suited the study.

Grounded theory has four fundamental criteria to ensure the appropriate application of theory to phenomenon.

- Fit- describes the realities under study in the eyes of the subject.
- Understanding- explains the major variations in behaviour in the area.
- Generality- if it fits and has understanding the grounded theory has achieved generality.
- Control- the theory provides a conceptual framework elucidated in a structured empirical method, it can be described as having control.

- (Glaser and Strauss, 1967).

The method of theory generation was a constant comparative analysis. This is an inductive and deductive process, best explained as a cyclical analysis from the general to the particular. Generating data, analysis of data, comparison with a priori knowledge, re-generation of data and formulation of theory to explain the themes or codes emerging from the data. Constant comparative analysis is collecting and analysing data simultaneously, it requires data collection, categorising codes in respect of emerging concepts and identifying core categories. The method involves returning to the field cyclically to eventually produce a theory. The constant comparative method was achieved in this study by constantly returning to the data, moving between open coding and axial coding, comparing codes with categories, categories with sub-categories and constantly cycling between these areas. This constant cycling allowed me to engage fully with the emerging data and to provide concepts to explain phenomenon.

Coding is a process by which data are analysed, conceptualised and re-formulated in previously unidentified ways. This process is fundamental to the whole generation of grounded theory. The procedures of grounded theory are designed to:

- Build a theory, not test a hypothesis.
- Ensure the research process is rigorous.
- Help researchers overcome biases and assumptions that can be introduced to the research process.
- Provide the grounding needed to develop rich, explanatory theory that relates to the reality it represents.

(Strauss and Corbin, 1990).

The coding system in grounded theory incorporates three sets of coding procedures to assist the researchers to dissect the data, conceptualize it and re-build it in new ways (Priest et al, 2002). These three coding phases are termed open coding, axial coding and selective coding.

Open Coding

Open coding is the first phase of the analytical process involving fracturing or taking the data apart and analysing the data for differences and similarities (Strauss and Corbin, 1990). Data refers to sentences or paragraphs of transcripts of speech from interviews. Examples of questions the researcher should consider when analysing the data should include; what is the basis for this point of view? Do other participants hold this belief or similar? Is there any relation between themes or concepts? These questions were constantly being asked throughout the research process and as the researcher I was constantly being drawn into debate with the data as to what formed a particular opinion and why. The aim of open coding was to define concepts that form units of analysis. The list of concepts was sorted into groups of related phenomena to become categories.

The interview transcripts were examined to totality, to obtain an overall sense of the content and a flavour of the responses by the participants to various issues. Each transcript was read several times to enable me to engage with the emerging data. Coding began with a sentence-by-sentence, word-by-word analysis. As the data were presenting some of the words or phrases appeared meaningful and these were highlighted. These highlighted words or phrases were labelled by the use of memos and written on index cards. The words or phrases were not allocated any interpretation at this stage. Strauss and Corbin (1990) suggest the use of in vivo codes to avoid early interpretation of the emerging data. These codes are a direct representation of the words used by the participants.

Initially there were a total of one thousand one hundred and seventy four in vivo codes; many of these codes were repeated throughout the six transcripts, examples of open codes from participant one can be observed in appendix 9. Similar codes were amalgamated and index cards were used to identify sub-categories linking codes with similar codes. The index cards were moved re-moved and grouped and re-grouped until sub-categories emerged that seemed fit the codes that were produced. I visited the data on a daily basis for a prolonged period to enable me to filter the data and the sub-categories. There were a total of twenty-three sub-categories on completion of the open coding. The sub-categories translated into concepts by amalgamating groups of ideas or sub-categories. This notion advances open coding to the next phase axial coding.

Axial Coding

Axial coding in contrast seeks to compare and connect categories and sub-categories. This phase seeks to identify rationale to define categories, such as conditions that influence phenomenon and to contextualise the data (Strauss and Corbin, 1990). Strauss and Corbin use the terms context, conditions and consequences to analyse the emerging phenomenon. The researcher must consider the context in which the phenomena occurred, what conditions were present and what the consequences of the actions that arose. At this stage as patterns in the data emerge, it is possible to generate tentative hypotheses or make statements of similarities and differences between the emerging phenomena.

The process of amalgamating sub-categories and codes was commenced tentatively at the beginning of the analysis. The process as stated is a constant comparative method and referring to the codes sub-categories and memos, I began to link sub-categories with concepts or ideas that encapsulated the amalgamated sub-categories and codes. The categories that were produced encapsulated the open codes represented more abstract definitions of the sub-categories. Sub-categories were allocated to categories as they emerged and seemed to describe the resultant data. This was a very challenging stage of the research process, as decisions I made were my own responsibility and as a result of my own plausible interpretation of the emerging data. Six categories emerged on completion of the axial coding process. The categories although linking the data, were distinct and separate entities with properties incorporated by the codes and sub-categories.

Selective Coding

The objective of selective coding is to discover core categories to which all categories have a relation. The researcher identifies the main theme from the emerging categories. The core category has six essential characteristics:

- It recurs frequently in the data.
- It links data together.
- It explains much of the variations in data.
- It has implications for a more formal or generalised theory.
- As it becomes more intense it advances the theory.
- It permits optimal variation in analysis.

(Strauss, 1987)

This final phase is the most challenging aspect to grounded theory as it seeks to integrate codes, as opposed to many studies proposing to be grounded theory, merely presenting themes. Selective coding makes alterations and integrates codes and categories into a true grounded theory (Priest et al, 2002). The limited time frame and the small sample size prevented the progression to the selective coding process.

The process of grounded theory was eloquently presented by Hutchinson and Wilson, (2001) in the form of a flow chart (appendix 2). This diagram shows clearly the process from primary review of the background literature to contextualise the research question to the positing of a theory. This particular model informed this study and aspects of the model were adhered to, given time constraints and the small scale of the study. What I did not do was to produce a basic sociological and psychological process or achieve selective coding, due to the small scale of the study and the time limitations. The secondary literature review was conducted following the analysis of the findings to provide theoretical sensitivity and place this study in context with existing knowledge relating to the understanding of the constituents of the therapeutic relationship.

Memos

To induce a grounded theory the analysis of data must be elicited at a theoretical level. Memos should be a part of this procedure to apply principles of constant comparative analysis, in the form of index cards, journal recordings or on a computer to establish connections between the data. The emphasis is related to identifying ideas or concepts. Ideas are identified and can be recalled with ease due to the code or codes that they describe with each memo (Strauss and Corbin, 1990). Questions the researcher needs to ask when memoing include:

- Are they separate codes?
- Is one code a property or a phase in another?
- What are the conditions that influence a code?

Through repeated questioning of memos and codes a theory is developed. The basic sociological psychological process emerges and the data becomes integrated. The conditional matrix forms a pictorial representation of an analysis of levels of the world and society we engage with. The picture is presented as a set of circles with the inner circle concerned interactions most closely related (actions pertaining to the phenomenon. The outer ring represents issues pertaining to an international level (issues such as international politics or governmental regulations). The conditional matrix has various levels between these extremes including national, community, organisational/ institutional, group or individual and interaction level. The conditional matrix as described by Strauss and Corbin (1990) was conducted in this study in the form of contextualising the data within national and international psychiatric nursing, however the basic sociological and psychological process was not fully extrapolated due to the small scale of the study.

Rigour

The pursuit of excellence in research is referred to as rigor; this involves accuracy, discipline and adherence to detail. Within the naturalistic paradigm certain steps should be taken to ensure scientific rigor. Sandelowski (1986) describes four aspects of trustworthiness promoting rigor within the naturalistic paradigm. These four criteria refer to credibility, applicability, consistency and confirmability. These four principles of trustworthiness have been upheld throughout the research process.

Credibility

The credibility of the study is increased when scholars and readers of the study identify with the phenomena having read the study. Recording of the interviews was the first step to maximize credibility, this action ensured that all the data were collected and no information was lost. The data and the interpretations were presented to two of the participants to verify the findings. The two participants were asked to comment on the accuracy of the stated categories, in addition two psychiatric nurses independent of the study were asked to comment on the findings of the study. Feedback from these individuals can be observed in appendix twelve. Member validation is a process to check the information presented is accurate and that varying perspectives are encountered (Seale, 1999).

Consistency

The audit trail of the researcher is an important consideration to ensure consistency of the study. Consistency from this study would be clear if another scholar would find similar results from the same data given similar circumstances (Sandelowski, 1986). I attempted to make explicit my decision trail by stating a rationale informing all decisions. This transparency extends to decisions relating to participants, data collection and analysis. Appendix eleven describes the decisions made during the research process and provides evidence to support the claim that the study is consistent and other researchers would have made similar decisions.

Confirmability

Confirmability in this study refers to the research loop described by Sandelowski (1986), returning to the participants to verify results. In addition the confirmability is reinforced in this study by the production of research notes made during each interview (appendix 10) and the transparency of the decision trail. Notes were taken during each interview to assist in the data collection process and to assist in the data analysis.

Applicability

Guba and Lincoln (1994) posit that the notion of applicability is confirmed when the hypotheses can be transferred between contexts depending upon the degree of fit, that describes the realities of the study in the eyes of the subject (Glaser and Strauss, 1967). Candidates who volunteer to participate in research projects are often the more articulate and informative, a treat to applicability can occur when members of a population are not well represented (Sandelowski, 1986). This study incorporated a purposive and volunteer sample and therefore the sample is a fair representation of the population.

Ethical Considerations
Ethics are concerned with issues of right and wrong, good and bad and doing no harm. In research ethical consideration must be maintained at all stages of the process. During this study the researcher has been cognizant of the ethical principles and these have been applied throughout the study. Thuroux's five principles apply these principles to a research scenario and are applied under similar forms as follows:

- Value of life
- Goodness and rightness
- Justice and fairness
- Honesty
- Individual freedom

Cited in Tschudin, (1995)

When undertaking research in social sciences, particularly a nursing study, cognizance must be given to a possible role conflict between, the nurse as an advocate and the nurse as a researcher.

Ethical approval to conduct the study was sought from the Director of Nursing and Regional Manager. The aim of the study was to involve psychiatric nurses and, as cited by Bell (1993), approval from authorities governing nurses is sufficient to gain ethical approval. A full informed consent procedure (appendix 4) was completed by each participant and a copy informed consent form was enclosed to the Director of Nursing and Regional Manager, in addition to a letter requesting ethical approval (appendix 5). Reply (appendix 8). A coding system was used to maintain anonymity and this was conveyed and made explicit to the participants in the form of informed consent.

Confidentiality was considered in relation to ethical considerations; it is based on the right to anonymity and linked to the ethical principle of the respect of person. Informed consent was given in the light of the following and could be withdrawn at any stage of the research process:

- Clarity of the purpose of the study and justification.
- Description.
- The benefits.
- The risks.
- Right to withdraw.
- Confidentiality.
- Who to contact for further follow-up.

(Polit and Hungler, 1995)

Responsibility for disclosure or maintenance of confidentiality rests with the individual moral agent. There can be no breach of confidence if information is not regarded as confidential or secret and is already in the public domain. A coding system was utilized in the research. Confidentiality was maintained throughout the entire research and it was explained to each participant that the results of the study will be presented in the form of a dissertation and this is alluded to in the informed consent procedure (appendix 4).

This chapter described a range of methodological aspects in relation to this investigation. Issues relating to research paradigms and how this study is located in relation to the naturalistic paradigm were discussed. A rationale for the choice of research methodology informed, by this research paradigm was described. The research method chosen was discussed in detail, including data collection and data analysis methods. Ethical considerations were discussed and an explanation of how these principles relate to this investigation given. Chapter four that follows gives details of the findings of the study. The final chapter then discusses in detail the research analyses.

REFERENCES

Annells M. (1996) Grounded theory method: philosophical perspectives, paradigm of inquiry and postmodernism. *Qualitative Health Research.* 2, 4, 375-391.

Bell J. (1993) *Doing your research: A guide for first time researchers in education and social science.* Milton Keynes, Open University Press.

Benzies KM. and Allen MN. (2001) Symbolic interactionism as a theoretical perspective for multiple method research. *Journal of Advanced Nursing.* 33(4), 541-547.

Blaikie N. (1993) *Approaches to social enquiry.* Cambridge, Polity.

Blumer H. (1969) *Symbolic interactionism: perspective and method.* Englewood Cliffs, NJ, Prentice-Hall.

Crotty M. (1998) *The foundations of social research: meaning and perspective in the research process.* London, Sage.

Glaser BG. (1992) *Basics of grounded theory analysis: emergence vs forcing.* Mill Valley, California, Sociology Press.

Glaser BG. and Strauss A. (1967) *The discovery of grounded theory: strategies for qualitative research.* New York, Aldine de Gruyter.

Goffman E. (1961) *Asylums.* New York, Doubleday Anchor.

Guba EG. and Lincoln YS. (1994) Competing paradigms in qualitative research. In: *Handbook of Qualitative research* (eds Denzin NK. and Lincoln YS.), pp 105-117. London, Sage.

Hutchinson SA. and Wilson HS. (2001) Grounded theory: the method, In: *Nursing research: A qualitative perspective, 3rd edn* (ed Munhall PL.), pp 209-243. London, Jones and Bartlett.

Keats DM. (2000) *Interviewing: a practical guide for students and professionals.* Buckingham, Open University Press.

Mason J. (1996) *Qualitative Researching.* London, Sage Publications

Maykut P. and Morehouse R. (1994) *Beginning Qualitative Research: A philosophic and practical guide.* London, The Falmer Press.

Mead GH. (1934) *Mind, self and society.* Chicago, University of Chicago Press.

Morse JM., Solberg SM., Neander WL., Bottoroff JL. and Johnson JL. (1990) Concepts of caring and caring as a concept. *Advances in Nursing Science.* 13(1), 1-14.

Norton L. (1999) The philosophical bases of grounded theory and their implications for research practice. *Nurse Researcher.* 7(1).

Paley J. (2000) Paradigms and presuppositions: the difference between qualitative and quantitative research. *Scholarly Inquiry for Nursing Practice: An International Journal.* 14,2.

Polit D. and Hungler B. (1995) *Nursing research: Principles and methods, 5th Edn.* Philadelphia Pa, Lippincott.

Priest H., Roberts P. and Woods L. (2002) An overview of three different approaches to the interpretation of qualitative data. Part 1: theoretical issues. *Nurse Researcher.* 10, 1, 30-42.

Ritzer G. (1996) *Sociology theory, 4th edn.* New York, McGraw Hill.

Sandelowski M. (1986) The problems of rigor in qualitative research. *Advances in Nursing Science.* 8(3), 27-37.

Schumacher K. and Gortner S. (1992) (Mis)conceptions and reconceptions about traditional science. *Advances in Nursing Science.* 14(4), 1-11.

Seale C. (1999) *Researching Society and Culture.* London, Sage Publications.

Stern PN. (1994) Eroding grounded theory. In: *Critical issues in qualitative research methods* (ed Morse JM.), pp 212-223. Thousand Oaks, CA, Sage.

Strauss A. (1987) *Qualitative data analysis for social scientists.* Cambridge, Cambridge University Press.

Strauss A. and Corbin J. (1990) *Basics of qualitative research.* Newbury Park CA, Sage.

Treacy MP. and Hyde A. (1999) *Nursing Research Design and Practice.* Dublin, University College Dublin Press.

Tschudin V. (1995) *Counselling skills for nurses, 2nd Edn.* London, Baliere Tindall.

Chapter Three

FINDINGS

This Chapter describes in detail the findings of the study and presents the research results systematically using grounded theory methodology. It begins with a brief description of procedural issues relating to the study. A description of participants involved in the study follows, including a rationale for their inclusion. This is followed by a presentation of the findings by discussing the analysis of the emerging data. The findings are presented in categories and sub-categories. These findings are a plausible interpretation of the data, it is not a definitive interpretation, as previously discussed naturalistic inquiry has many interpretations of reality. The findings are not generalisable; however they do represent the views of the participants involved in the study.

DESCRIPTION OF PARTICIPANTS

The participants in the study were six psychiatric nurses employed in various areas of the psychiatric nursing service in a region in the South of Ireland. The sample nurses were generic psychiatric nurses with no post registration training in counseling or related courses that could bias the results towards the discipline of counseling. The research refers to psychiatric nurses' perceptions of the constituents of the therapeutic relationship; these perceptions could have been biased by additional training in counseling.

The sample of psychiatric nurses was composed of post registration nurses with between two and ten years experience. The assumption is that nurses trained over two years will have sufficient exposure to form an educated opinion on the topic of interest. The ten-year threshold is identified due to; nurses trained beyond this period would have been educated in a different curriculum. The six nurses were equally divided between the genders.

Results

The results of the study outline the perceptions held by psychiatric nurses in relation to the therapeutic relationship. The categories that emerged are formed by the opinions of the participants. The categories are related; to how psychiatric nurses combine a therapeutic role with a service provision role, how the process of therapy is identified in practice, how do psychiatric nurses learn to develop therapeutic relationships, time is an important influence on the success or failure of the therapeutic relationship, what skills are required to form therapeutic relationships and how attitudes affect the formation of therapeutic relationships. The findings of the study are presented in the form of categories and sub-categories that emerged from the data.

SCHEMATIC REPRESENTATION

The following section discusses the data supplied by the participants of the study and provides context to the data. This process is best summarized in the form of a schematic matrix. The matrix contextualizes the data and as indicated by Strauss and Corbin (1990) it provides a theoretical framework to produce findings. The framework begins with professional or role conflicts, indicates the processes necessary to develop therapeutic relationships, examines how learning occurs, examines the nature of time limitations and culminates in the influences personal and attitudinal factors affect the development of the therapeutic relationship.

Nursing is Providing a Service

This category is comprised of five sub-categories relating to the dichotomous relationship between therapy and the provision of psychiatric nursing services. The five sub-categories are; professional aspects of care, individualized care, working in a team, the helping aspect is based on a caring approach and the nature of the therapeutic relationship is dependent upon illness and class. The category suggests that the diversity of psychiatric nursing results in a 'jack of all trades-master of none' scenario. Psychiatric nurses have so many tasks and duties to perform that, to perform any task to the optimum results in detracting from another area.

Category	Sub-category	Context
Nursing is providing a service.	Professional aspects of care.	Psychiatric nursing is an activity located in a professional role; how does this affect the therapeutic relationship?
	Individualized care.	Psychiatric nurses espouse individualized care; is this possible and how does it affect the therapeutic relationship?
	Working in a team.	The participants of this study highlighted that psychiatric nursing is mostly performed in teams; positive and negative aspects of this are discussed.
	The helping aspect is based on a caring approach.	Providing help or care was an aspect of the psychiatric nurses' role highlighted by the participants.
	The nature of the therapeutic relationship is dependent upon illness.	The degree and type of intervention is governed by the psychiatric condition of the patient.
The process of therapy.	The impact of personal life issues.	Personal issues have an inevitable influence on how and why therapeutic relationships are formed.
	Therapeutic framework.	What guides practice and how do relationships begin, develop and end?
	Therapeutic factors.	What is therapeutic? What makes it different from any other relationship?
	Curative factors.	How do people cope and what changes circumstances to enable this coping?

		Dependency levels.	The normalizing process decreases the dependency on nurses. How does this influence the therapeutic relationship?
Learning in the therapeutic relationship.		Experiential learning.	How do psychiatric nurses learn to develop therapeutic relationships?
		Intuitive learning.	
Developing therapeutic relationships is limited by time.		Incremental nature of the therapeutic relationship.	To develop a relationship with an individual in any therapeutic sense takes time. How is this compromised by the psychiatric nursing role?
		The nurses' minute.	Often psychiatric nurses have to prioritize workload. How does this impact on the therapeutic relationship?
		Role diversity.	Psychiatric nursing is very diverse and has many demands.
Skills required to form therapeutic relationships.		Trust	
		Humor.	
		Conscious decision making.	Skills identified by the participants of the study.
		Providing information.	
Attitudes.		Therapeutic boundaries.	How do psychiatric nurses compromise therapeutic distance and professional boundaries?
		Different personalities.	How do personality conflicts affect the development of the therapeutic relationship?
		Non-judgmental attitude.	Does this exist? Is it possible in psychiatric nursing?

PROFESSIONAL ASPECTS OF CARE

This sub-category indicates that psychiatric nurses have a responsibility to conduct themselves in a certain manner. This manner is dictated by a code of conduct augmented by personal morals and ethics.

> You feel somewhat obliged to help your clients. You're there, they are there for help. You should be in a position to help. You have knowledge. You are part of a profession (P 4.3).

This professional aspect of care relates to how psychiatric nurses change their approach within relationships and what makes these relationships professional and therapeutic. Therapeutic relationships differ from any other kind of relationships due to the fact psychiatric nurses are bound by a code of conduct and also a duty of care.

> But with regard to professional, again it comes down to that balance of getting as close as you can to a patient but keeping your distance (P3.2).

This statement indicates that the involvement between patient and nurse is close enough to develop a therapeutic role and distant enough to remain within the professional code of conduct and preserve the altruistic, professional and caring nature of the relationship.

> It is a relationship that is a professional relationship that you would build up with a patient. You can't get too close or too friendly. But there again you don't want to be cold and too hard on them. You have to find a balance of the friendly side of it but yet the side where you have to have an element of control and discipline with the patient...It is hard to find a balance with some patients. With psychiatry, you get a lot of manipulative patients that will try and manipulate you through getting really friendly with you and trying to evade getting personal with patients. Keeping it professional is important (P3.1).

These professional aspects of care sometimes restrict the nature of therapeutic interventions. The professional responsibilities interfere with the natural, maturational development of relationships in terms of therapeutic endeavor.

> Take for instance someone with a personality disorder a lot of their behavior is attention seeking and what you want to say to them is to get a grip, but you can't say that because it is not professional (P2.2).

The sub-categories detailed in this section indicate that psychiatric nurses are often called upon to make decisions in the patients' best interest. These decisions are often in conflict between are therapeutic rationale and the provision of care in a professional sense. This dichotomy between therapy and service provision affects how psychiatric nurses engage in therapeutic relationships.

INDIVIDUALIZED CARE

This sub-category relates to the approach psychiatric nurse have towards patients and how they treat each patient according to their needs. This treatment is dictated by how nurses identify patient needs and approach this treatment in different ways.

> ...they are all different. They are all very much totally different from one another. All their needs are different as well. I suppose somebody might need a bit of help or somebody to listen to or chat to and somebody might not need that at all (P5.3)

Individualized care in relation to how psychiatric nurses perceive the therapeutic relationship also describes a process of care provision in relation to continuous care by a team of nurses. Continuity of care is significant in relation building therapeutic relationships, due to the relationship development being beyond the control of the individual nurse.

> ...staffing levels play a lot in it. I think it definitely does. To a certain degree, it must affect the relationship. You have a patient that is looking at you from admissions and saying right this is my man in here. If I have anything wrong, I will go to this man. If anything is bothering me, I go to this man. You come down the road two days later and he comes up to you and you say 'look I'm not actually dealing with you. Dr. x is dealing with you today. That is John's job, go and talk to John'. John has to start two days later to build up a relationship with the patient. And John could only be on it for a day or two, and then it is somebody else (P3.5).

As indicated by these codes individualized care is possible in theory; however continuity of individualized care is harder to achieve. In relation to the therapeutic relationship the implication is that the relationship building is staccato and inconsistent.

Working in a Team

As indicated nursing on the whole is an activity performed in teams, inter-disciplinary teams and multi-disciplinary teams. The result is that any therapeutic relationship developed is dependent, not only on individualized factors, but also factors between individuals and between disciplines. This sub-category describes the relationship between teamwork and developing the therapeutic relationship. The notion of responsibility and the degree nurses feel empowered within the multi-disciplinary team significantly affects the development of therapeutic relationships.

> In so far as giving care to the patients, my part in the multi-disciplinary team is kind of limited in ways, in so far that I'm not allowed opinionate things. It's limited in ways I find it is only a personal thing that you are still kind of answerable to doctors (P3.1).

In any therapeutic scenario the therapist would exhibit a degree of unconditional positive regard, but this theory is exposed when describing relationship development and teamwork. Personality difficulties and ability to develop rapport is compromised when the psychiatric nurse is involved in a particular method of care delivery. Primary nursing for example, in a real sense, involves nurses working with a group of patients, but the degree of choice and development of rapport is questionable.

> You are working with a certain sector or doctor and you have those clients and that is it. You have no choice. There is going to be personality clashes (4.4).

The positive aspect of teamwork is illustrated by the learning that is undertaken by psychiatric nurses from and between nurses. Psychiatric nurses would describe learning their role predominantly experientially. Traditionally psychiatric nurses have learned their role by clinical placements augmented by 'block periods' in a school of nursing. This study as previously stated is undertaken with this cohort of traditionally trained nurses and reflects this phenomenon.

> ...when you have your colleagues that are working with you as well, if there's problems happening needless to say you can ask somebody what they think, what they would do, or can you help me out with this one (P5.4)

The Helping Aspect is based on a Caring Approach

The nature of nursing is presented at times as a helping or caring profession. The codes identified in this sub-category support this statement. The sub-category presents codes relating to how nurses have a role to help others.

> ...this is my job, I love it...so the relationships I form here they need help, they need help in some shape or form. They need help, you have help to give them (P1.3)

Nursing in general, but particularly in psychiatry is dominated by the desire to help or care for fellow human beings. This altruistic notion is of course diluted by the personality traits and attitudes of the individual nurse.

> Some people make better nurses than others. I think there has to be an element of care in every nurse. There has to be some element of wanting to help people (P4.3).

Helping or caring is the domain of psychiatric nursing that historically has been the area most emphasized when psychiatric nurses describe their role. It is however the area possibly least studied empirically and other disciplines have provided the evidence to support practice. This evidence does not easily translate between disciplines, as psychiatric nursing is a specific discipline with specific aspects forming the role.

The Nature of the Therapeutic Relationship is Dependent upon Illness and Class

This sub-category describes how the development of the therapeutic relationship is dependent upon the nature of the patients' illness or disorder. The type of illness in conjunction with individual factors mitigate to impact on the formulation of the therapeutic relationship.

> ...it's just that if somebody was psychotic or quite paranoid you might approach them differently. That somebody elated say or quite depressed you'd take more of a slower approach with them or may be more of a one to one (P1.1).

In addition to types of illnesses or disorders encountered in psychiatric nursing, patients are representatives of various social strata. The sociological influences upon individuals also affect the nature of the therapeutic relationship.

> If you dealing with a solicitor or doctor, which I suppose we all have at times, I suppose you are not going to speak in the same way as you are to somebody who has not received a full education. So language-wise, you try and bring yourself to their standard as you perceive it without talking down to certain people or talking up to others...You put it into basic kind of terms, if you are trying to explain illnesses or problems they may have. As in you'd feel a bit high rather than tell them they are in a manic phase (P4.4-5).

Psychiatric nursing is perhaps unique in relation to forming relationships determined as therapeutic. This unique situation is manifested by the requirement to form relationships with patients who on occasions have been admitted to hospital involuntarily.

> The other side of it is hard in acute psychiatry to build up a relationship with a patient is when you have temporary admissions. And then, turn around and try and develop a nurse/patient relationship with them (P3.6).

The sub-category emphasizes that psychiatric nurses on occasions have to form therapeutic relationships with people who may not have anything in common with the nurse, or the person has been entered into the therapeutic milieu under duress.

The contradiction between therapy and service is summarized by a professional accountability, responsibility to the public and providing a service; balancing with the necessity to develop a close yet distant and individualized relationship. It seems by the evidence supplied in this study that the balancing of these factors are inextricably linked and are opposing phenomena.

THE PROCESS OF THERAPY

This category describes the way therapy is fluid and transient and the factors that distinguish a therapeutic relationship as opposed to other relationships developed in people's lives. The process of therapy is dependent upon a number of factors and these are reflected in the five sub-categories that are incorporated in this category. These five sub-categories are; the impact of personal life issues, therapeutic framework, therapeutic factors, curative factors and dependency levels.

The Impact of Personal Life Issues

This sub-category describes the affect personal feelings, prejudices personalities and attitudes have on the forming of therapeutic relationships. Psychiatric nurses are professional people however they are people, with the same expressions of emotions and feelings as the people they are treating. This is reflected in confusion in relation to the degree of personal experiences they should or should not express to the patients. The question is; would my experiences burden the patient further or would an insight into handling the situation in a different way benefit the patient?

> ...the emphasis of the relationship is on the patient, you allow them to deal with issues that they want to deal with without burdening them (P4.4).

The confusion extends to an ability to express in an articulate way the difficulty of therapeutic boundaries and clearly locating themselves within this relationship.

> ...when I said distance earlier on I meant as in not distant as in physical distance, I meant closeness as in I'd never discuss my private life with a patient (P1.6-7).

The role of a psychiatric nurse is to treat patients who have psychological illnesses and disorders of the mind. Part of this treatment is to enable the patient to develop life skills to cope with life events. What needs to be borne in mind is that in addition to being patients and staff the relationship is a more intimate relationship.

> ...you are a person and they are a person... (P2.5)

This more intimate relationship is reflected in the expression of parity in a relationship and respecting the professional aspect of the care relationship.

> ...I'm only human, I'm a human being at the end of the day and we all have our ups and downs in work, we have maybe bad days in work, good days in work and in your personal life as well... (P1.5).

This sub-category indicates the difficult decision psychiatric nurses need to make in relation to the type and extent of personal information they divulge to patients to enhance the therapeutic nature of the therapeutic relationship. These decisions are made in relation to professional aspects of the nurses' role and taking account of personal morals.

> Bridges could be built an awful lot quicker if you were going to be very open about who you are, what you do, as in where you come from, you know, personal situations...I just think myself I would hold back on any information outside work. I feel that it doesn't need to come into the patient/nurse relationship (P5.7).

This sub-category emphasizes that although psychiatric nurses aspire to bracket personal life influences it is at times impossible to disown life experiences. These life experiences significantly influence how psychiatric nurses develop therapeutic relationships.

Therapeutic Framework

This sub-category describes how the therapeutic relationship develops and how psychiatric nurses can and do formulate a loose plan to address forming these relationships. These frameworks are not formally recognized structures but are personal plans that individual nurses adopt to give structure to their everyday practice in relation to forming therapeutic relationships.

> ...you know, I'd always introduce myself, shake their hand in situations where you can do that you know, I'd never be stand offish with a patient, if they'd let me sit in the chair beside them you know, kind of go through their property with them...I'd always talk through what I was going to do with them as well. (P1.6)

The frameworks nurses adopt are based on good mannerly behavior that any individual may adopt on meeting a person for the first time. The difference between any mannerly individual and a psychiatric nurse is the extent the nurse goes to, to enable the individual to 'feel at home' or 'feel comfortable' with their illness or disability.

You initially introduce yourself and bring the patient to a quiet environment where you can speak without interruption. Sit down face to face, just try and speak calmly and let them know what is happening, what the next steps are.

Maybe do something simple like offer them a cup of tea to help them feel more relaxed. And then once you see that they are starting to relax, initiate more conversation on their problems. The best thing to do in a therapeutic relationship is to explain (P2.2-3).

The framework of therapeutic intervention is a loose expression of how each nurse controls their practice and gives a degree of structure to an everyday activity. This framework is an individual expression of their practice and becomes so second nature even to describe it is difficult.

Therapeutic Factors

This sub-category describes the participants' perceptions of what factors are therapeutic in the therapeutic relationship and how these relationships differ from other relationships. These factors are a combination and collection of factors described as contributing to a therapeutic scenario. The first code describes the nurse's role in providing care to needy individuals.

> …caring for somebody who can't provide it for themselves (P1.8).

Therapeutic factors within therapeutic relationships relates to how the patient reacts to the interventions offered by the nurse. This reaction is typified by the notion of a rapport between the patient and the nurse. The rapport refers to the affinity and emotional closeness between two individuals and how this is recognized and used in a therapeutic way.

> …a rapport you can develop with the patient (P1.1).

The affinity and closeness between nurse and patient is only a portion of the relationship, other aspects include, what nurses do with the information gleaned in the therapeutic milieu. The relationship between nurse and patient must be a relationship held in confidence to enable the patient to feel confident in sharing their inner world, this was one of the clearer aspects understood by the participants. This understanding may be due to the fact nursing and therapy share the common notion of confidentiality.

> …therapeutic and confidential relationship. You have to be non-biased (P2.1).

The participants in this study recognized that nurses at times need to be advocates for patients and make appropriate decisions for the patients. The nurses also need to make authoritative decisions and act in the patients' best interest, which at times causes conflict.

> ...control and discipline with the patient (P3.1).

Therapeutic factors identified in this sub-category are the perceptions of the participants of the study. The factors described indicate the factors necessary to engage, sustain and develop a positive change in the patient.

Curative Factors

This sub-category differs slightly from the previous sub-category in relation to the level and degree of permanency in lifestyle changes and coping with illness or disorder.

> Our role is to help people get better. Our role is to make their life as comfortable as possible (P4.1).

A notion in therapeutic relationships that is reflected in this study is the notion that to cure a patient in psychiatric terms is a misnomer and that the illnesses displayed by patients are managed or coped with. When describing curative factors in this study I am referring to a change of circumstances for the patient to improve their condition. This improvement can be as a result of a lot of factors and this study is interested in the improvement attributed to the therapeutic relationship. One of the curative factors identified by the participants of the study was an interpersonal statement reflecting the personality differences and how this affects the improvement that patients make.

> You will either draw somebody out of themselves or you won't (P5.1).

Nurses often don't acknowledge their abilities or achievements but some of the participants of this study recognized that they do have a significant role to play in the improvement of the patients' conditions.

> We have some answers; we don't have all the answers (P2.2).

The curative factors outlined in this sub-category identify what positive change may be made in the patient and how the psychiatric nurse acts as a change agent. The codes identified by the participants describe the role of the nurse in this change and the role of the patient.

Dependency Levels

This sub-category describes the relationship between nurse and patient and how this relationship changes as the patient becomes 'better' and more able to deal with their illness or disorder. The nurses' role in this scenario is to enable the patient to understand the facets of their disability and enable them to cope better. The therapeutic relationship is the vehicle to drive this process and the end product is normalization and a return to independence.

> ...they need to conduct their normal day to day living then when things start back on the increase they slowly regain their independence you know for themselves where they come in they might be more dependent on nursing staff, even on medication or something you know where they felt that they needed to use that as a crutch but as they progress in their mental health or as the recovery process progresses their become more independent. (P1.9).

Recognition of this normalizing process is the marker to indicate the therapeutic positive movement or change. It is vital for the psychiatric nurse to recognize this positive development in the patients' recovery process, as this is an indication that the therapeutic process is therapeutic or not. The relationship between nurse and patient changes as the therapeutic process progresses and it is subtle change from a dependent relationship to a more shared relationship.

> ...they are moving from a stage of dependence to independence, and part of that process is that the relationship becomes more equal, from being one-way to being more of a shared process (P4.8).

The process of therapy therefore is a progressive cyclical relationship with the emphasis on understanding from the point of view of the nurse and the patient. The patient needs to learn how to deal with whatever ails them. The nurse needs to understand how the patient improves to enable them to reproduce similar therapeutic processes in the future. These change processes are both professional and personal factors that influence the connection between patient and nurse.

LEARNING IN RELATION TO THE THERAPEUTIC RELATIONSHIP

How psychiatric nurses learn to practice is a significant factor in reproduction of appropriate methods to treat patients. If we understand how learning was produced we can amend future learning to tailor psychiatric nursing practice with the hindsight gained through examination of current trends. Two forms of learning were identified in this study, reflected in two sub-categories: experiential learning and intuitive learning.

Experiential Learning

This sub-category describes how psychiatric nurses learn aspects of their role through a process not necessarily formal, but just as pervasive as the formal curriculum. This process of learning experientially is driven by a natural curiosity of the person learning. It stems from the motivating factors intrinsic to each individual learner. These motivating factors are described in the codes and relate to practical, social, personal and research problems of interest to the psychiatric nurse.

> ...learned about forming therapeutic relationships, it was through observing what other members of staff were doing, tailoring your own processes and learning and putting that into action yourself, based on what you had observed. So it wasn't anything you learned academically in the school (P5.4).

In relation to learning about the therapeutic relationship and how this is located in the role of a psychiatric nurse, this process is a socialization process that involves all learning, both formal and informal. This process of learning from an experiential point of view is displayed by participants in the study constantly referring to learning their role by watching, absorbing and adopting aspects of how senior colleagues perform their duties.

> ...you would watch other nurses and see how they relate to patients and you would pick up how some people don't relate very well and how some people relate very well. And you get tips from more experienced staff...(P2.1)

> ...the therapeutic relationship is a very real thing, it is between two people. It is very different to read about and put it on a piece of paper. It is more of an experience based, almost an apprenticeship (P6.5).

This sub-category describes the participants' opinions of how they learn to form and develop therapeutic relationships. The sub-category describes learning through experience and how this learning is incremental and practical experience of the therapeutic relationship.

Intuitive Learning

This sub-category describes how psychiatric nurses sometimes act on instinct as opposed to any learned methods. The learning involved in intuitive caring is in the form of life experience in combination with experience collected through exposure to the role.

> ...after a few years of working, you start to pick up on non-verbal cues. You start to see things that maybe, of course they are not always there, but that you think there is something going on with the client which you just feel isn't the same as it was the day before. Maybe their mannerisms have changed...that sixth sense that kind of, that there is something there that they are not the same as they were the day before maybe... (P4.2)

Psychiatric nurses appreciate that they must behave within accepted standards but have difficulty explaining with any degree of coherence what this process is or how decisions are reached informing this behavior.

> I mean you have your own intuition which I would call it your gut instinct...intuition if you were in a situation and you kind of thought there was something just not right (P1.7)

The intuition described therefore by the participants is an application of human skills by a knowledgeable professional. The application of skills developed through a socialization process within the remit of a professional nurse.

> ...I gathered a body of knowledge about subjects that I use in my professional life, which I use in liaison with interaction skills. The human skills are the foot in the door and then I proceed to try and pass across the information... I could have human skills and no knowledge to back it up and it

would be pretty useless, or I could have huge knowledge and no human skills (P6.5).

Intuitive learning is significant in relation to how psychiatric nurses develop skills, this sub-category describes how the participants of this study learned to develop and utilize knowledge and skills relating to the therapeutic relationship. This learning is described as intuitive, but different interpretations of the meaning of intuition are expressed.

DEVELOPING THE THERAPEUTIC RELATIONSHIP IS LIMITED BY TIME

Time in relation to any therapeutic intervention is crucial and to identify how much time is allocated to these activities in psychiatric nursing is difficult, due to the diversity of role function. In any other therapeutic relationship, outside the discipline of psychiatric nursing, time is negotiated and it forms a crucial part of the contractual arrangement with the patient. This category explores the affect time can have on forming and maintaining therapeutic relationships in psychiatric nursing. The category is made up of three sub-categories describing the participants' interpretation of how time influences the therapeutic relationship; namely the incremental nature of the therapeutic relationship, the nurses' minute and role diversity.

Incremental Nature of the Therapeutic Relationship

This sub-category describes how forming the therapeutic relationship takes time and it is important that the nurse realizes the timing process. The participants in this study showed that the timing of interventions depends on the relationship factors and illness factors and these are very much individualized.

> …if they come into hospital in the evening time or you know that they're too distressed and upset and tearful and anxious and angry and all the kind of emotional aspects that comes with an admission to hospital but think it's from the next day from like when they're reviewed the next day when they're calmed down a little bit when the realization hits…(P1.5)

The difference in interpretation of how long it takes to form therapeutic relationships is interesting. Participants had different views about how long it takes to form effective relationships; however this maybe reflects the difference between different personalities and different interpersonal skills development.

> A relationship isn't going to develop within twenty minutes, an hour or a day even. It does take at least three or four days to build up a genuine good relationship with a patient, in so far as they trust you (P3.2)

This sub-category emphasizes that the development of the therapeutic relationship does not happen immediately and requires time to develop. The participants of this study describe the therapeutic relationship being built and factors in the relationship being cumulative.

The Nurses' Minute

This sub-category illustrates the emphasis on genuineness and openness in the relationship between nurse and patient. This genuineness is emphasized by the way in which the nurse performs his or her duties and how this is conveyed to the patient. For example, if a nurse states they will do a particular task for a patient, this task is performed and not forgotten due to this prioritization process.

> The nurses minute again, getting back to that. That you do have time for them even though you have twelve other clients or whatever it is, that you do make certain time for certain people during the day. If they ask you to do something, you do it. That you don' do it the next day. If you are writing reports or a care plan at the time, that you can put it down for a few minutes at least (P4.5)

This sub-category emphasizes that nurses often have to priorities use of their time. The participants of this study expressed a willingness to be genuine to the patients by fulfilling stated tasks. There is a realization however that this is not always possible and prior tasks are a priority.

Role Diversity

The profession of psychiatric nursing is multi-facetted as indicated previously and the nurse is drawn in many directions. This sub-category indicates how the many and different roles impact on the forming of the therapeutic relationship.

> ...quite often you would feel you don't have enough time to give to patients because you have so many other things to do. You have, like, you now take on students as preceptor. There are so many other jobs you have to do and you are often caught short-staffed as well, so you don't always have the time for patients that you would like to have and you find yourself saying that I'll come back to you and you're hoping you will have the time to come back to them but you don't always have the time. But you can priorities. You know, sometimes people say we have to make the beds or we have to do things that aren't as important as sitting down with a patient. Some things can wait, so you just have to prioritize (P2.3).

The category indicates the importance of time constraints on the development of therapeutic relationships and how the participants of this study perceive these constraints. The loose formation of contracts between the nurse and the patient is an important pre-requisite for the development of therapeutic relationships.

SKILLS REQUIRED TO FORM THERAPEUTIC RELATIONSHIPS

Skills involved in forming therapeutic relationships require interpersonal skills that can be learned but the learning tends to be in the form of learning about oneself. The field of counseling and psychotherapy have embraced this principle, psychiatric nurses are however more reluctant and describe this as detracting emphasis from the needs of the patient. This category describes the interpretation the participants have of skills required to form therapeutic relationships. The category is made up of four sub-categories illustrating what participants perceive to be skills required to develop therapeutic relationships. These sub-categories are: trust, humor, conscious decision making and providing information.

Trust

This sub-category indicates that psychiatric nurses place a huge emphasis on the development of trust and feel that the skills required to form a trusting relationship are understated. The first aspect of the trusting relationship is enabling the patient to feel safe and secure and how this is conveyed to the patient.

> ...build the trust over a period of time but if the patent doesn't get a sense of kind of security and safety when they come in or that they can't confide in you, you know you're missing out on a whole, kind of, you know, therapeutic sense where they might feel they can't engage with you or they wont ventilate if they've any concerns...(P1.1).

Conveying safety and security to the patient is important and equally important is the ability to convey understanding of the patients' point of view. The participants of this study refer to this understanding as empathic understanding. The ability to put oneself in the other persons' shoes is important when trying to treat a person with respect and dignity.

> You have to look at it from the patients' point of view, they are expecting something from you. They are expecting you to be able to help them (P2.2).

Sometimes acting as a confidante and listening to the patient is sufficient to enable the patients to unburden themselves and feel less isolated in their despair. This ability to allow the patient ventilate their despair is often referred to in nursing reports, but the skill is more intricate than merely listening. It is a process enabling the patient to feel the centre of attention and to listen to what they are telling you without passing judgment. If this can be achieved the patient will develop trust and be able to rely on the nurse.

> I suppose if a patient confides in you, you must have done something right in their eyes. They found in themselves to approach you and confide in you (P3.9)

If the nurse can convey trust in the form of safety and security, empathic understanding and acting as a confidante then the therapeutic relationship will be enhanced and the relationship said to be therapeutic. These factors need not be present in any other form of relationship and are specific to the therapeutic nature of psychiatric nursing relationships.

> Basically, being a confidante, doing what's right for a person you are dealing with and having their best interests at heart. Being honest (P5.2).

This sub-category indicates that trust is an important component in developing therapeutic relationships. The participants of this study clearly emphasize developing a trusting relationship would enhance a therapeutic outcome.

Humor

An understated skill that most psychiatric nurses have is the ability to use humor as a means of developing relationships with patients. This use of humor has rarely, if at all, been recognized as a feature in psychiatric nursing practice. However this sub-category clearly illustrates that participants in this study utilize humor in various ways and for varying reasons. Firstly the use of humor to develop a pathway to engage further with the patient and make them feel at ease.

> …well it helps to sit down and make them comfortable and to sit in front of the person and use eye contact. To smile at them I suppose. Maybe if you could even make a little joke it would help them relax as well (P2.4).

The use of humor enables the relationship to be more inclined towards the friendly relationship as opposed to the professional relationship that was discussed previously. Humor assists in the development of rapport and the collapsing of any hierarchical restrictions to the therapeutic nature of the relationship.

> I think it makes it easier and the relationship is formed quicker if the person is outgoing and able to chat away, or crack a joke and have a banter beforehand (5.11).

The relationship between nurse and patient initially involves interpretations and misinterpretations. The feelings experienced by patients are based on past experiences and media expressions of the nurses' role. Participants in this study differentiate between the friendly relationship and the authoritarian relationship and associate the development of a therapeutic relationship with friendliness and the use of humor as a vehicle or skill to achieve the therapeutic relationship.

> I find joking with them works an awful lot better rather than being serious with them. You know, having a friendly relationship rather than an authoritarian one (P4.4).

The role of a psychiatric nurse is to deal with stress and tension expressed by patients every day. Participants expressed the view that a bit of humor can at times diffuse difficult situations and clear the air, particularly when patients are experiencing stress or anxiety provoking situations.

> ...a smile or wink or even a bit of black guarding. Even cracking a small joke eases the stress and the tension (P5.9).

This sub-category, although on the surface, describes the use of humor as a positive and beneficial activity that most of the participants would describe as ice-breaking, diffusing or increasing friendliness. The reverse can be true and the use of humor can be belittling and demeaning, particularly between nurses. For example jokes about patients between nurses with no malice intended but an undertone of mocking the patients.

Conscious Decision-Making

This sub-category indicates how the participants of this study perceive their role in relation to the development of therapeutic relationships in terms of a conscious decision making process. The scope of professional practice for nurses indicates that nurses should perform their duties within their sphere of competence. The participants in this study questioned whether or not they perform this particular aspect of their role consciously or not.

> ...it's kind of a conscious effort or whether I do it naturally I think I always kind of if somebody comes in, more so with the obviously female patients (P1.6).

Nursing in general is an activity that is performed in the spur of the moment with nurses reacting to situations and these reactions are based on how they reacted previously and how they were taught to react. This results in nurses often having to 'talk to themselves' to stop and think before reacting.

> I think you often have to stop and think before you actually say something or before you make plans on the care of the patient. You really have to stop and think which would be the right way to go and you have to maybe involve other people, other members of the team, before you make a decision (P2.2).

> You have a professional distance as well. You have to have some distance in yourself and stand back and look at the situation differently (P6.2).

This sub-category indicates that although developing relationships with patients and with people in general is a natural process. The development of relationships in a therapeutic sense is a more conscious process.

Providing Information

This sub-category relates to the way nurses have an educative role and patients are sometimes looking for advice (maybe to affirm what they think anyway). Giving advice or providing information is tricky; how do nurses know the advice they are giving is good advice. Participants in this study described giving information in a factual way about unequivocal topics such as what processes the patient will be undergoing.

> You would always be conscious of explaining what you are going to do for a patient and learn them to ask questions. To give them the answers when they ask questions, not to be fobbing them off. Try to give them answers as close as possible (P2.3).

The communication process is the giving of a message and the reciprocal returning of that message. This communication process in psychiatric nursing as described by the participants in this study is described as a more informal process, with a hidden agenda of giving and gaining information.

> I think people are more forthcoming with information when they are not asked directly. You probably get a truer picture and you can actually assess them by just chatting and asking them the same questions but in a more conversational typesetting (P5.11).

In addition to the type of information given to patients the clarity of the delivery of the information is important. This code emphasizes the importance of how the information is conveyed to the patient.

> Simple short sentences, certainly initially. People have difficulty sometimes in taking in information, especially in a stressful time, like an admission to hospital or suffering from an illness (P6.4).

This category describing skills identified by the participants reflects how the communication process is utilized in a more understanding and understood relationship. The human relationship is about social animals in social settings behaving appropriately. In this study it is identified that this human behavior is produced in a therapeutic setting and if a degree of trust and rapport is evident then the relationship will flourish, if it is not it will perish. These skills are shown to be life skills as opposed to any learned or professional skills.

ATTITUDES AFFECTING THE DEVELOPMENT OF THE THERAPEUTIC RELATIONSHIP

This category describes the different attitudes that patients and nurses may have and how these attitudes impact on the therapeutic relationship. The category is divided into three sub-categories namely: therapeutic boundaries, different personalities and non-judgmental attitude. These sub-categories reflect the personality difficulties nurses and patients experience, how nurses try to bracket these difficulties and what a therapeutic distance means. Psychiatric nurses involved in this study identified these attitudinal factors as affecting the development of helping relationships.

Therapeutic Boundaries

This sub-category illustrates the confusion that exists in relation therapeutic distance or how close a psychiatric nurse feels they can become engaged with a patient. This closeness or distance is governed by the individual personalities involved and the degree of professionalism exhibited by the nurse.

> ...it comes down to that balance of getting as close as you can to a patient but keeping your distance. They don't need to know a lot of personal information about you. The best way is get as close as you can and build up a good enough relationship with a patient that they trust you. Keep your professional distance from them, without getting too familiar with them or anything like that (P3.1).

The relationship is developed on the basis of what the patient requires, and is patient focused. The participants in this study felt the need to detach themselves from the relationship in relation to keeping a professional boundary. Maintaining these boundaries is necessary to maintain an emotional distance between nurse and patient, to ensure appropriateness of behavior.

> But in the therapeutic relationship, there is a kind of distance and a barrier that you don't cross...that is purely to help the patient, purely to keep that detachment there. It is not there that you don't open yourself up to them. You don't want to throw your problems as well back on the patient (4.3)

Maintaining therapeutic boundaries in the formation of the therapeutic relationship results in mutual respect by the patient and the psychiatric nurse. This mutual respect is based on that fact that the nurse respects the difficulties the patient may be experiencing and the patient respects the attitudes and skills the psychiatric nurses displays.

> ...when you are in work, I think you have to maintain some degree of, I won't say standing back or not getting too close to somebody, because I think you have to have, I won't say respect for each other but, there has to be some level of boundaries (P5.5).

This sub-category reflects the opinions of the participants of this study in relation to how close or distant the patient and the psychiatric nurse are required to engage in the therapeutic relationship

Different Personalities

This sub-category presents the participants views relating to how personality differences or difficulties can impinge on the development of therapeutic relationships. The first code presents the view that the psychiatric nurse must bracket opinions or biases formulated in their own lives and treat the patient on face value.

> You have to talk to yourself before you go into the patient and tell yourself you have to approach them in a certain way. You can't be judgmental towards them. They are coming for help, they are coming into your care. You have to remain professional no matter what your opinion is (P2.5).

In this sense, by bracketing their own personality traits or learned prejudices the nurses are betraying their own personality and presenting an artificial front to the patient. This is contrary to the formation of therapeutic relationships, in the sense that, there is a requirement in a therapeutic sense to be genuine in forming relationships with patients.

> You would be more inclined, I think, to leave a patient ventilate a little bit more than you would with your friends...You would leave them get so far, certainly further than you would with your friends...(P4.4)

The attitude of the nurse plays an important role in how a patient perceives their involvement in the relationship. The nurse's personal history, professional development or personal maturity may impact on the development of the relationship.

> As a child I would have been very, very open. A lot of it wouldn't even be job specific, in that my own personality would be somewhat open and perhaps I fit my personality around the job. I don't think you can take on the persona of a nurse (P6.4).

Factors of the nurse's personal and professional life influence the way their personality is formed. In addition the degree of job satisfaction and burnout would affect the degree of involvement or degree of interest the nurse has in their job and hence the involvement with the patient.

> I think a lot of it has to do with personality as well. If you have somebody who has no interest as well and will probably just gauge someone with the bare minimum and see what has to be done. I think patients pick up on that too. Whereas if you have someone who is happy in what they're doing. Maybe some of it can be learned, maybe some of it is who you are to a certain extent. Maybe some people find it easier to get in on a conversation than others (P5.8).

This sub-category indicates that to engage in any therapeutic relationship the personality differences and difficulties affect this engagement.

Non-Judgmental Attitude

The attitudes of the nurses and the patients were discussed previously in this study; however one specific attitude that was mentioned on a number of occasions by numerous participants was a non-judgmental attitude. This sub-category is significant in relation to how nurses hold personal opinions and do not act or display these opinions to the patient.

> Just say if a patient came in that I'd never - to me attitude means non-judgmental in kind of hand in hand that's to me I'll never judge a patient no

matter what situation they came in no matter how much it bothered me or annoyed me or whatever, you'd never let that show when you're dealing with a patient (P1.7)

The participants were at variance in describing the affect personal opinion or attitudes affect the development of the therapeutic relationship. Some participants' described being able to successfully detach themselves from these attitudes when dealing with patients, other participants felt that non-judgmental attitude is a fallacy that nurse can never detach themselves from attitudes developed over their lifetime. Opinions about individuals are formed from the very moment the nurse meets the patient and this is an unavoidable natural result of human inquisitiveness.

> To a degree, you can be non-judgmental but a lot of people, and I suppose it's human nature, you make up a small part of your mind on someone on appearance, which is wrong. You look at someone, oh, he could be such and such. And you look at another person and you say he looks nice, he could be pleasant. You know, you shouldn't, but you do. I won't say you 100% make your mind up on appearance alone, but it does go a small part of it (P3.8).

> ...you can't be non-judgmental because everyone makes decisions about people every second of every day. You don't act on your judgments or certainly your personal judgments shouldn't affect your professional behavior (P6.5).

This category illustrates quite clearly that the attitudes that patients hold and the attitudes that nurses hold affect the development of any relationship, but particularly the forming of therapeutic relationships. These attitudes are formed through life experience and are so pervasive that to even abandon them for a temporary period is challenging for the professional psychiatric nurse.

In this chapter I have attempted to present a plausible explanation of the information gleaned from semi-structured interviews in relation to the participants' perception of the constituents of the therapeutic relationship. The findings presented are an interpretation of views expressed by six psychiatric nurses. The method to analyze the data was a grounded theory approach as defined by Strauss and Corbin (1990). The key categories identified in the study were: how the process of therapy is identified in practice, how do psychiatric nurses learn to develop therapeutic relationships, time is an important influence on the success or failure of the therapeutic relationship, what skills are required to form therapeutic relationships and how attitudes affect the formation of therapeutic relationships. The following and final chapter is an analysis of the findings in relation to a priori knowledge. Strauss and Corbin (1990) refer to this process as theoretical sensitivity, taking account of existing literature, personal and professional factors to synthesize the study to existing knowledge in relation to the therapeutic relationship.

REFERENCES

Strauss A. and Corbin J. (1990) *Basics of qualitative research.* Newbury Park CA, Sage.

Chapter Four

DISCUSSION

The following chapter will endeavor to amalgamate the findings of this study with the evidence supplied in the available literature relating to the constituents of the therapeutic relationship in psychiatric nursing. The study objective was to explain how psychiatric nurses perceive the therapeutic relationship fits their role and what the relationship is comprised of. The previous chapter described the findings of the study. This chapter will be structured around the six categories identified in the findings. One comment of note is that due to the small scale of the study, tentative hypotheses are made; however the positing of a theory would be unreasonable. What the study does however is highlight the interpretations of the participants and compare these interpretations to what is described in the literature.

REVIEW OF THE FINDINGS

The findings of the study identify the perceptions held by psychiatric nurses in relation to the therapeutic relationship. The categories described the views of the participants in relation to; to how psychiatric nurses combine a therapeutic role with a service provision role, how the process of therapy is identified in practice, how do psychiatric nurses learn to develop therapeutic relationships, time is an important influence on the success or failure of the therapeutic relationship, what skills are required to form therapeutic relationships and how attitudes affect the formation of therapeutic relationships.

The first thing to recognize from the study is the identification of how the therapeutic relationship is located in the role of a psychiatric nurse. Barker (1998) and Peplau (1962) described the therapeutic relationship as the essence of the psychiatric nurse. If the essence or crux of psychiatric nursing is the development of therapeutic relationships between psychiatric nurses and patients, research must clearly identify the components of such relationships. It is difficult to identify these components due to a number of factors involved, the two main factors being the convolution of variables involved and the assumptions relating to the location of therapeutic liaisons within the role of psychiatric nursing. The participants in this study however quite clearly identify the therapeutic relationship as one of the many diverse roles of the psychiatric nurse. This therapeutic relationship role is identified as an intervention, the fact that it is imperative that nurses engage in therapeutic relationships is none the less a facet of their role. This theoretical position is supported in the literature by Gournay (1996) who views psychiatric nursing as incorporating the role of developing therapeutic relationships within their overall psychiatric nursing role.

Nursing is providing A Service

The first category identified in this study described psychiatric nursing as providing a service to the public and patients. The role of a nurse is first and foremost to provide a service to the patients and the public in general. Part of this role as stated is to develop therapeutic relationships. These relationships are therapeutic due to the patient requiring help from a state of despair and the professional nurse has an onus to provide this service or care. The problem of the nurse providing this service is that the psychiatric nurse has so many functions to perform that to provide therapy within a relationship is ultimately so time consuming and intricate that the nurse can not fully commit to the therapeutic relationship. The fundamental premise as described by Fealy, (1995) is that a professional nurse develops a caring relationship with a client/patient, as determined by organisational dictums and professional codes of conduct, assuming the person being cared for has an illness, crisis or unable to care for themselves. The role of the psychiatric nurse as described in this study highlights the fact that all nursing is performed in teams of some shape or form, whether multi-disciplinary or inter-disciplinary teams. This emphasizes that psychiatric nurses have responsibilities primarily to the patients, but also have responsibilities to fellow nurses and nursing students. In relation to forming therapeutic relationships this is significant, as indicated by the findings of this study in relation to how nurses learn to develop therapeutic relationships. The requirement to form therapeutic relationships as indicated in this study is described therefore as a balancing of therapeutic factors and the provision of a nursing service.

Stickley (2002) describes the role of the psychiatric nurse and discovers that psychiatric nurses are in a profession that is demanding and insufficiently trained to perform that role. This is significant to this investigation as one of the questions raised relates to the degree psychiatric nurses develop therapeutic relationships consciously and competently. Having stated that the dichotomy exists between therapy and service provision and how this impacts on how and why psychiatric nurses develop therapeutic relationships, it is still an important role of the psychiatric nurse to engage in therapeutic relationships. The following section describes the process of therapy and how this process is dependent upon numerous factors.

The Process of Therapy

LM. Weibe (University of Toronto, Toronto, unpublished dissertation) determined that connection in the therapeutic relationship is the experience of sharing a subjective world. Connection within the therapeutic relationship relates to the degree to which the patient and the nurse become engaged and it is grounded in the relationship in which it exists. Therefore, the experience of connection in the therapeutic relationship is unique. In this study the cyclical nature of the therapeutic relationship is explored and the participants would concur that the connecting features and the process of therapy is dependent upon personal and professional factors. The mutual work of therapy is connecting, as is the interactive process of building the therapeutic relationship.

Five types of therapeutic relationship were conceptualised by Clarkson (1994) these types of relationships were reflected in the responses by the participants in this study. These responses concurred with Clarkson (1994) that differing approaches needed to be taken at different times to different problems.

The working alliance she describes as an agreement between carer and patient formulated to address a mutually agreed objective. The participants in this study would agree that some common goal is warranted, however the process mitigated against the formulation of a contractual arrangement. What exists in the majority of cases is a common goal that is loosely stated between nurse and patient. The developmentally needed relationship is described as initiating a corrective or informative function, during which identification of maladaptive interpersonal relationships are addressed. This study highlighted that the psychiatric nurses in this study identified a clear role in relation to providing information to patients. This role was separated into the type of information and the method of delivery. The I-Thou or person-to-person relationship is formed upon the subjective experience of the carer and the therapeutic essence is the product of the relationship itself, providing a forum for ventilation of experiences and emotions.

Marmor (1982) identified seven elements described as change producing; these were identified within the frame of this study, but expressed more explicitly by the following elements:

- The formulation of a relationship determined by real and fantasised qualities of carer and patient.
- The expression of emotional tension.
- Learning or development of understanding.
- Operant conditioning based on approval or disapproval and corrective responses during the therapeutic experience.
- Suggestion and persuasion, overt and covert.
- Development of self-awareness.
- Repeated reality testing and reflection.

(Marmor, 1982)

Rowan (2002) describes three approaches to therapeutic liaisons, instrumental, authentic and transpersonal. The instrumental approach is universal as a way of being; it is learned responses or developmental material that is reinforced by socialization agents such as the family or mass media. The findings of this study indicate that the participants of this study recognize that learning about the therapeutic relationship is an experiential process fuelled by the natural curiosity of the individual nurse. The authentic approach requires some kind of initiation, which is quite readily acquired through therapy. The initiation of some form of intervention is as a result of a professional duty of care. The participants of this study would confirm this view and most stated that nursing is dominated by the desire to help and if this was not the case people would not enter nursing. It involves dealing with certain closed or subconscious aspects of existence, all those aspects of ourselves that we are initially reluctant to recognize. And the transpersonal approach also needs some kind of initiation, which has to be acquired through some of spiritual practice. It has to be some form of practice that teaches us, on an experiential level, that our boundaries are uncertain, that we do not live totally in isolation. It informs us that we are fundamentally divine, not limited by a narrow definition of our humanity. The learning of the therapeutic relationship is explored in more detail in the following section and illustrates from the literature supplied by the participants in this study that it is akin to a socialization process.

Learning in Relation to the Therapeutic Relationship

Participants in this study identified two forms of learning or understanding how to form and develop therapeutic relationships. The participants on the whole described learning about the therapeutic relationship through a socialization process. Numerous studies have been conducted in relation to the socialization of nurses indicating that socialization factors are powerful and pervasive (Davies, 1993, Gerrish, 2000, Gray and Smith, 2000, Philpin, 1999). All these scholars conclude that the socialization experiences of nurses affect clinical practice irrespective of educational experiences shaping practice. The participants in this study would confirm that most of the learning in relation to developing therapeutic relationships is conducted in the form of a socializing process. Experiential learning or the socialization process is described by the participants in this study as a process of developing skills by participant observation. Experience and intuition it that sense are interlinked but are also separate identities. Carper (1978) first described ways of knowing in nursing and legitimized different forms of knowledge and development of knowledge. Heath (1998) drawing on the theories of Carper described intuitive knowledge as an accumulation of past experiences by the expert nurse who get to the heart of the problem. The participants in this study refer to gut instinct at times governing decision-making and action plans. Pyles and Stern (1983) also identified the importance of clinical experience in the development of gut feelings and suggested that intuition was an integral part of comprehensive patient care.

Altshul (1972) postulated the development of therapeutic relationships between nurse and patient was the result of intuition and not a consciously competent theory driven process. Therefore if the essence of psychiatric nursing is the development of therapeutic relationships and these interactions are as a result of intuition, ergo psychiatric nurses are neither utilizing evidence based practice nor are they performing their therapeutic role within the scope of professional practice. The evidence shared by the literature and the participants of this study suggest that intuition is a combination of experience and personal knowing (Carper, 1978, Pyles and Stern, 1983, McCutcheon, 2001). Intuition is therefore a skill that affects the effectiveness of the therapeutic relationship and intuition must be acknowledged in the scope of practice and its use documented.

Developing the Therapeutic Relationship is Limited by Time

The role of the psychiatric nurse as stated previously is diverse and due to the service provision aspect they are pulled in many directions. This factor alone necessitates a prioritization of the use of time. As stated by the participants in this study the priority the majority of the time is to provide care. Boykin and Schoenhofer, (1993) proposed the notion or philosophy of caring as a nurturing process and caring reflects the human mode of being. The basis of this philosophical perspective is extended from the works of theorists, such as Roach (1984) concurrent with the view that caring is a human experience and a reflection of morality and the ethical principle of respect of the person.

They view the act of nursing as a reaction to needs and maintain that nurses are caring individuals whose assignment is to promote health and welfare, through caring actions. It is also stated that similar to Roach, (1984) caring is not exclusive to nursing, however, caring is a unique expression within the profession of nursing.

Tickle-Dengen (2002) upon reviewing the available research suggested that communication functions within therapeutic relationships are fundamentally formulated in three concurrent and interlinked stages. These stages are the development of rapport, the development of a working alliance and maintenance of the working alliance. These stages appear to be formed similar to the map of counseling espoused by Burnard (1994). The participants in this study identified that no formal process or framework exists to formulate the therapeutic relationship. This process is individual and depends upon time with no formal contracts.

Due to the fact that developing the therapeutic relationship is incremental in nature, do nurses have time to formulate these relationships? The conclusion drawn in this study is no; due to time restrictions, the diverse role, the impact of personal factors, the affect of illness and the affect personality difficulties have on forming these relationships. Having stated the difficulties psychiatric nurses face in their everyday encounters with patients and prioritization, the following section describes the skills necessary to develop therapeutic relationships. The literature assumes that nurses have skills and time to formulate therapeutic relationships (Barker, 1998, Burnard, 1994, Marmor, 1982, LM. Weibe, University of Toronto, Toronto, unpublished dissertation). This study emphasizes that psychiatric nurses do not have time or the appropriate skills to competently develop therapeutic relationships.

Skills Required to Form Therapeutic Relationships

Participants in this study are at variance with the available literature (Rogers, 1981, Burnard, 1994, Marmor, 1982). The skills developed and utilized in therapeutic relationships is an application acquired human skills accompanied by knowledge of how to intervene when patients are in distress. The ability to develop these skills is individual and an expression of the personality and moral development of the individual and not a demonstration of skills acquired through any academic exercise. Humanistic psychology that influences nursing curricula emphasizes that interpersonal skills can be learned (Heron, 1974). These skills however relate to intervention skills identified in the six category intervention analysis (Heron, 1974). These intervention skills are part of how the therapeutic relationship is performed. Participants in this study identify intervention skills and personal and professional development as key components to competently form therapeutic relationships. One point of note was the regularity the participants of this study stated that the use humor was a skill that they used in their day-to-day interventions with patients.

The use of humor in the therapeutic relationship was a common feature identified by most of the participants of this study. The use of humor was felt to be a skill most psychiatric nurses possess. Humor was described in this study as a pathway to further dialogue, assisting in the development of rapport, a therapeutic tool to alleviate stress and devolving the professional relationship to a friendly level. Most of the participants of this study felt the use of humor benefited the relationship in some way. Sayre (2001) would not agree with this position, in a study of 59 psychiatric nurses she identified two forms of humor used by psychiatric nurses, whimsical and sarcastic. Sayre (2001) identified that psychiatric nurses engaged more in sarcastic humor and suggested that recognition of detrimental effects of joking behaviors should be an area of concern. The participants in this study remarked on the beneficial effects of joking behaviors, but this was from the perspective of the nurse and untested from the perspective of the patient.

Therapeutic interventions are described as caring actions undertaken by nurses such as, attentive listening, teaching or educating patients, touch, presence, technical competence or indeed all interventions to promote health and well-being (Morse et al, 1990). Techniques or skills identified as being fundamental to formulating, sustaining and advancing the therapeutic relationship are generally accepted to fall into listening, questioning, encouraging ventilation, reflecting on content and clarifying (Minishull, 1982, Burnard, 1994). The literature therefore would suggest that the development of the therapeutic relationship is founded on trust (Burnard, 1991, Rogers, 1981, Tschudin, 1985); this was a feature of the findings of this study.

Attitudes Affecting the Development of the Therapeutic Relationship

The successful formulation of the therapeutic relationship is dependent upon attitudes peculiar to the individual therapist. Attitudes adopted will depend to some extent on the particular therapist and their training in interpersonal skills. Rolfe (1990) argued that the theorist most carers associated with identification of attitudes is the theories of Rogers (1981). He identified three essential attitudes namely, genuineness, respect and empathy. However Omer (2000) would argue against this general conception stating that desirable attitudes in relation to the formulation, exploration and sustaining of therapeutic relationships have no universal correct application. The findings of this study would lean towards agreeing with Omer (2000) as the diversity, complexity and individuality of psychiatric nursing and in particular the therapeutic relationship mitigates to form therapeutic relationships on a day-to-day individualized basis.

Empathy, warmth, and the therapeutic relationship have been shown to have more impact in relation to patients' perspective or therapeutic effect than more specialized or technical interventions (Lambert, 2001). Decades of research indicate that the provision of therapy is an interpersonal process in which a main curative component is the nature of the therapeutic relationship. This study indicates that participants were at a loss to clearly articulate a meaning for non-judgmental. Although all the participants stated that to form therapeutic relationships psychiatric nurses needed to be non-judgmental, some felt that being non-judgmental was a misnomer. This position was formed by the notion that their own developmental psychology influenced prejudices that were so pervasive that being non-judgmental was not possible.

Limitations

The objective of the study was to examine in more detail the constituents of the therapeutic relationship, to this end the objectives were realized, however no research is entirely flawless (Sandelowski, 1986). This particular study although examining the phenomena in detail only examines the question from a nursing perspective. The therapeutic relationship is a reciprocal relationship and no account is given from the patient perspective. This position is partly as a result of the limited time frame to conduct the study. The study is also limited in the type of methodology utilized, as the findings are not generalisable to a larger population (Mason, 1996). However the findings are of significance as these opinions cited by the participants are supported by a priori knowledge. The study is also limited due to the fact that it was a small-scale study and the researcher a novice researcher. The study is also limited by the size of the sample; due to the sample being small the research selective coding process and the basic psychological and sociological process could not be completed.

The study was limited by the fact interviews were the method of data collection; ideally a combination of interviews and observation would be a better way to affirm the findings (Field and Morse, 1985). In relation to the study findings what was not addressed which is of significance was the notion of measuring the degree of therapeutic change.

As previously stated the purpose of the study is to extract meaning from an activity that is undertaken by psychiatric nurses every day of his or her working life. However this activity as previously stated is a two-way reciprocal relationship and the study is addressing the phenomena from the psychiatric nurses' perspective. As previously stated, the nature of the relationship between mental health workers and mental health users is changing. Mental health users are actively encouraged to be involved and empowered in care provision. This changing dynamic necessitates further research beyond this study to ascertain the full picture incorporating the perspective of the patient.

RECOMMENDATIONS

The recommendations from the study are that:

For Research

- The study could be repeated on a larger scale.
- The study could be a pluralistic study to identify a tool to measure the degree of therapeutic change or improvement. For example the study could incorporate qualitative and quantitative methodology, enable measurement of change and analysis of perceptions.

For Practice

- The study could take into account the perspective of the patients to draw conclusions in relation to effectiveness of interventions.

For Managers

- Psychiatric nurses sometimes need direction and assistance to organize and priorities their care provision. The participants of this study identified the need to accept the therapy and service provision roles and to acknowledge the difficulty in fulfilling these roles completely.

For Clinicians

- Understanding the role of the psychiatric nurse is difficult, as it is such an individual activity, however psychiatric nurses need to be sure that what they are doing is both therapeutic and consciously performed. Further study into how psychiatric nurses are aware and consciously develop therapeutic relationships could benefit psychiatric nursing practice.

REFERENCES

Altshul A. (1972) A Study of interaction patterns in acute psychiatric wards. Edinburgh, Churchill Livingstone.

Barker P. (1998) The future of the theory of interpersonal relation? A personal reflection on Peplau's legacy. *Journal of Psychiatric and Mental Health Nursing.* 5, 213-220.

Boykin A. and Schoenhofer S. (1993) Nursing as Caring: A model for transforming practice. New York, National League for Nursing.

Burnard P. (1991) Acquiring minimum counselling skills. *NursingStandard* 5(46), 37-39.

Burnard P. (1994) Counselling Skills for Health Professionals, 2nd Edn. London, Chapman and Hall.

Carper B. (1978) Fundamental patterns of knowing in nursing. *Advances in Nursing Science.* 1(1), 13-23.

Davies E. (1993) Clinical role modelling: uncovering hidden knowledge. *Journal of Advanced Nursing.* 18, 4, 627-636.

Fealy GM. (1995) Professional caring: the moral dimension. *Journal of Advanced Nursing.* 22, 1135-1140.

Field PA. and Morse JM. (1985) Nursing Research: the application of qualitative approaches. London, Croom Helm.

Gerrish K. (2000) Still fumbling along? A comparative study of the newly qualified nurse's perception of the transition from student to qualified nurse. *Journal of Advanced Nursing.* 32(2), 473-480.

Gournay K. (1996) Schizophrenia: a review of the contemporary literature and implications for mental health nursing theory practice and education. *Journal of Psychiatric and Mental Health Nursing.* 4, 441-446.

Gray M. and Smith L. (2000) the qualities of an effective mentor from the student nurse's perspective: findings from a longitudinal qualitative study. *Journal of Advanced Nursing.* 32, 6, 1542-1549.

Heath H. (1998) Reflection and patterns of knowing in nursing. *Journal of Advanced nursing.* 27)5), 1054-1059.

Heron J. (1974) The peer learning community. Guildford, University of Surrey.

Lambert MJ. (2001) Research summary on the therapeutic relationship and psychotherapy outcome. Psychotherapy: *Theory, Research, Practice,* Training. 38(4), 357-361.

Marmor J. (1982) Change in psychoanylitic treatment. In: Curative Factors in Dynamic Psychotherapy (ed Slipp S.), pp 60-70. New York, Magraw Hill.

Mason J. (1996) Qualitative Researching. London, Sage Publications

McCutcheon H. (2001) Intuition: an important tool in the practice of nursing. *Journal of Advanced Nursing.* 35(3), 342-348.

Minishull D. (1982) Counselling in psychiatric nursing Part 1.Nursing Times. 78, 1201-1202.

Morse JM., Solberg SM., Neander WL., Bottoroff JL. and Johnson JL. (1990) Concepts of caring and caring as a concept. *Advances in Nursing Science.* 13(1), 1-14.

Omer H. (2000) Troubles in the therapeutic relationship: A pluralistic perspective. *Journal of Clinical Psychology.* 56(2), 201-210.

Peplau HE. (1962) Interpersonal techniques: The crux of psychiatric nursing. *American Journal of Nursing.* 62, 50-54.

Philpin SM. (1999) The impact of Project 2000 reforms on the occupational socialisation of nurses. *Journal of Advanced Nursing.* 29(6), 1326-1331.

Pyles S. and Stern P. (1983) Discovery of nursing Gestalt in critical care nursing. The importance of the Gray Gorilla Syndrome. *Journal of Nursing Scholarship.* 15(2), 51-58.

Roach S. (1984) Caring: the human mode of being. Toronto, University of Toronto.

Rogers C. (1981) Client-centred Therapy. London, Constable.

Rolfe G. (1990) The assessment of therapeutic attitudes in the psychiatric setting. *Journal of Advanced Nursing.* 15, 564-570.

Rowan J. (2002) The three approaches to a therapeutic relationship: Instrumental, authentic, transpersonal. *Counselling Psychology Review.* 17(4), 3-10.

Sandelowski M. (1986) The problems of rigor in qualitative research. *Advances in Nursing Science.* 8(3), 27-37.

Sayre J. (2001) The use of aberrant medical humor by psychiatric unit staff. Issues in *Mental Health Nursing.* 22, 669-689.

Stickley T. (2002) Counselling and mental health nursing: a qualitative study. *Journal of Psychiatric and Mental Health Nursing.* 9, 301-308.

Tickle-Dengen L. (2002) Client-centered practice, therapeutic relationship, and the use of research evidence. *American Journal of Occupational Therapy.* 56(4), 470-474.

Tschudin V. (1995) Counselling skills for nurses, 2nd Edn. London, Baliere Tindall.

CONCLUSION

The results of the study indicate that the process of developing therapeutic relationships in psychiatric nursing is a combination of a learned experience through the acquiring of interpersonal skills; however these skills are redundant if the individual has not acquired sufficient life experience to intuitively appreciate the therapeutic aspect of the relationship. Intuition was a major feature of the findings from the study and the understanding of how this intuitive caring was learned was spurious. The constituents of the therapeutic relationship are clearly convoluted and interlinked with one aspect affecting and influencing the operationalisation of another. What is clear is that the skills, attitudes and knowledge learned in relation to the therapeutic relationship are learned through a socializing process or through experiential learning. This has significance in relation to forming a nursing curriculum, and in particular the assessment of clinical competence. The nurses need to develop these skills and demonstrate application of acquired life attitudes in the form of appropriate interventions. This demonstration can only be performed in the clinical area and therefore developed and assessed there also. The previous chapter examined the findings of the study and integrated these findings with the available literature in the field. The study identified components associated with the therapeutic relationship, as identified by the participants of this study.

As provided by the evidence in the literature interpersonal relationships and the therapeutic process within relationships has been the subject of discourse for approximately three decades. It is not coincidental that Peplau postulated her ideas at this time however consensus of opinion suggests that components formulating the therapeutic relationship have not been fully extrapolated.

What is clearly stated is the most appropriate research methodology is located within the interpretivist paradigm. If psychiatric nurses consider the positivist perspective to explore human experiences and relationships, may be a reflection of professional insecurity and as cited by Bevis (1982), nurses should be confident to utilize appropriate, but less favorable approaches to research to advance knowledge and nursing science. The question posed refers to perceptions of the constituents of the therapeutic relationship and the evidence supplied by the literature would indicate possibly the most appropriate method would be a grounded theory approach as the therapeutic relationship is a circumstance driven process. What the literature is also generating is a need to advance an epistemological basis for the exploration of professional practice and relate this issue to the impact on the clarification of the role of the psychiatric nurse.

The research also shows that psychiatric nurses are at times practicing at an intuitive level; this begs the question; are psychiatric nurses practicing what he or she espouses to practice or is it a paper exercise? The flip side of this scenario is that the therapeutic relationship is such an individualistic activity that some aspects of this relationship are described as immeasurable and need to remain such to allow spontaneity without measurement.

REFERENCES

Bevis EO. (1982) Curriculum Building In Nursing- A Process, 3rd Edn. St Louis, CV Mosby.

Appendix One

MAP OF COUNSELING

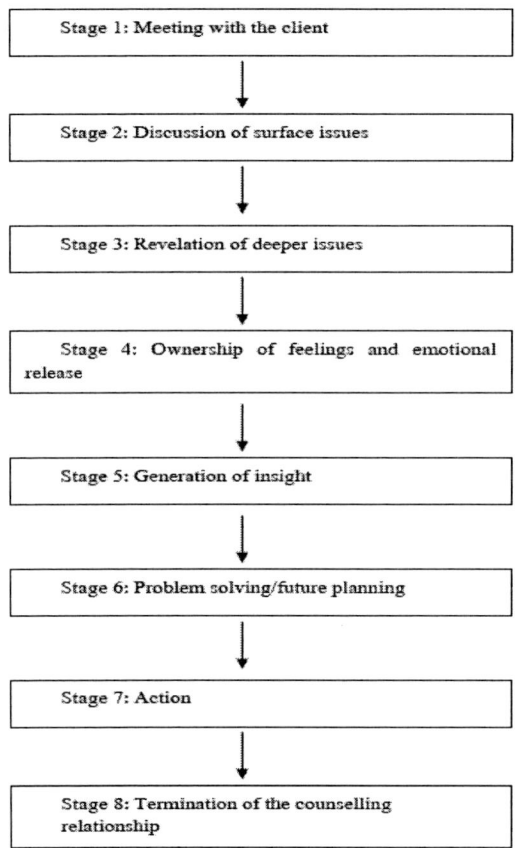

(Burnard, 1994)

Appendix Two

GROUNDED THEORY PROCESS

PROCESS	PRODUCT
Primary literature review	Discovery of sensitizing concepts, gaps in knowledge
Data collection: interviews, observations, documents	Masses of narrative data
Coding: coding paradigm, axial coding, constant comparative method	Level I codes- called in vivo or substantive
	Level II codes- called categories
	Level III codes- called theoretical constructs
Memoing	Theoretical and methodological ideas
Theoretical sampling	Dense data that lead to the illumination and expansion of theoretical constructs
Sorting	Basic social psychological problem and or process (BSP)-

	a central theme and/or basic social structural process (BSSP)- a central theme
Selective coding based on BSP, BSSP	Theory delimited to a few theoretical constructs, their categories and properties
Saturation of codes, categories and constructs	A dense, parsimonious theory covering behavioral variation; a sense of closure
Secondary literature review	Discovery of literature that supports, illuminates or extends proposed theory
Writing the theory research	A piece of publishable

(Hutchinson and Wilson, 2001)

Appendix Three

RESEARCH QUESTIONS/TOPIC GUIDE

SEMI-STRUCTURED DEPTH INTERVIEW

Warm up Questions

1) Please describe your role as a psychiatric nurse?
2) Where do you work?
3) What kind of patients do you nurse?
4) What do you understand by the term therapeutic relationship?

SOCIALISATION PROCESS

1) How did you learn about forming therapeutic relationships?
Learning- what learned Socialization?
When Intuition
How Academia

HOW CONNECTION OCCURS

1) How does this relationship differ from other relationships?
2) Are there any differences in how you feel?
3) Are there any differences in the way you think?
4) Are there any differences in the way you behave?

5) How do you go about developing the therapeutic relationship in your day-to-day practice?
6) Do you use a particular framework to guide you?

SKILLS IDENTIFIED/ USED TO FORM THERAPEUTIC RELATIONSHIPS

1) Could you describe skills you use in developing therapeutic relationships?

a) Language
b) Behavior

1) Where did you learn or develop these skills?
2) How did you learn or develop these skills?

ATTITUDES

1) How do attitudes affect relationship building?

a) Give examples of your own relationships
b) Previous experience-Individual
c) Previous experience-patient/knowledge

1) Do personalities affect forming therapeutic relationships?

IDENTIFY CURATIVE FACTORS

1) How do you identify positive therapeutic change or movement in the individual?
2) What factors are therapeutic in the relationships?
3) How do you know these factors are therapeutic?

Appendix Four

INFORMED CONSENT FORM - THERAPEUTIC RELATIONSHIP RESEARCH

1) *Purpose:* You are being asked to participate in a research study in which you will be asked to describe your thoughts, interpretations, perceptions and feelings as a practicing psychiatric nurse. The reason for conducting this study is to advance an understanding and develop a theory in relation to the constituents of the therapeutic relationship.

2) *Procedure:* The study will consist of 5-6 interviews that the investigator will conduct over a two-month period. The interviews will last approximately 60 minutes. You will be asked to respond to questions relating to your experiences in relation to utilisation and forming of therapeutic relationships. The interviews will be tape-recorded and the tape recordings will be erased once the tapes have been transcribed. At your request the interview may be terminated at any stage and the tape recorder turned off.

3) *Risks:* There are no anticipated physical risks involved by participating in this study. If you feel that the content of the interview is causing you feelings of stress or emotional discomfort please know that you may end the interview.

4) *Benefits:* There is no direct benefit to you for participating in this study. The results of this study, it is hoped, will assist psychiatric nurses to formulate a deeper understanding of what are the constituents of the therapeutic relationship and hence a more informed level of practice.

5) *Confidentiality:* Names will not be used in the reporting of any information you tell the researcher. All information that refers to, or can be identified with you, will remain confidential to the extent permitted by law. The study will be reported in a dissertation presented to University College Dublin.

6) *Participation is voluntary:* Your participation in this study is voluntary. If you decide to participate and later decide that you do not wish to continue, you may at any time withdraw your consent and stop your participation.

7) *Whom to contact for answers:* If there are any questions at any time regarding this study or your participation in it, you are free to consult with the researcher

8) I have read and received a copy of this informed consent form.

_____   _____

Signature of the researcher, date signature of participant, date

date_____

Appendix Five

Researcher
Address

17th February 2004

Director of Nursing
Address

> Re: Ethical approval to conduct research into what psychiatric nurses perceive to be the constituents of the therapeutic relationship.

Dear Mr.

I am seeking ethical approval as stated above. The research is proposed to involve 5-6 psychiatric nurses, with between two and ten years experience.

The study is proposed to be conducted as outlined in the enclosed informed consent form. The benefits and risks are explained to each participant.

I propose to utilize taped depth interviews of 60 minutes duration and the methods to conduct the research will be a grounded theory approach, as described by Strauss and Corbin (1997).

I would appreciate a reply as soon as possible to enable as much time as possible to analyze the findings.

I will make a copy of my research available when the research is complete.

Yours faithfully

Researcher

cc. Regional Manager, Special Hospital Programme, Address.

Appendix Six

Gant chart

Sep Oct Nov Dec Jan Feb Mar Apr May Jun Jul Aug Sep

Prelim reading ---------|

Lit review ----------------------------------|

Research Prop |------------------|

Ethical Approval |------|

Interviews (pilot) |----|

Interviews/field work |---------|

Transcribing |---------|

Open coding |

Axial coding Constant comparative analysis

Selective coding |

Analysis of data |----------------|

Writing up dissertation |-----|

Time line →

Appendix Seven

Resources and study management

The management of the research should include a timetable, citing a realistic agenda for the whole process, from conception or feasibility to completion.

Equipment needed would include:

- Computer
- Printer
- Office space
- Telephone calls
- Tape recorder and microphone
- Photocopier
- Paper and general stationary

General administrative costs are projected to include travel expenses, photocopying, telephone calls, paper, tapes, binding the study and printing.

Appendix Eight

Letter of Reply from the Director of Nursing Services

BF/JP

9th March 2004

Mr Adrian Scanlon

Re: Ethical Approval to conduct Research into what psychiatric nurses perceive to be the constituents of the therapeutic relationship

Dear Mr Scanlon,

I am in agreement for ethical approval to allow you to proceed with this research. I wish you well in your studies.

Yours sincerely

Director of Nursing

Appendix Nine

OPEN CODING- PARTICIPANT 1

CATEGORIES CODES COMMENTS

Attitudes affecting Not stand-offish Contradiction in emotional development of don't ever presume involvement

    TR. ALL GOOD INTENSIONS
    A distance
    Approach in different ways
    Closeness
    Sense of trust
    Warm feelings
    Make myself open
    Different personalities
    Never judgemental
    Respect privacy
    Non-judgemental
    Not take concerns lightly

Developing TR is Time specific: period of time
limited by time. Over a period of time
    Incremental
    nature of TR: needed sorting out
        realisation hits
        where to cut off
        patient begins to converse
        recovery process progresses
        TR working to its optimum

Individualised care. One to one
Converse freely
                Feedback
                Answer questions
                Limit setting
                Specialised needs- re-socialisation programmes
                 Personal hygiene programmes
                Talk normally- buzz words
                 my own kind of English
                 Psychiatry words
                own free will
                own way of working
                treat each intervention differently
                affecting their care
                plan in your mind
                admit that they have problems
                approach differently
                boundaries
                open conversation
                level like mates

    Trust safety and security: build trust trust staff links with
                            Actually come to me experience and
                            Rely on staff with you teamwork
                            In a vulnerable position
                            Building on a bit of trust
                    Confidence in you: confide
                            No one else to turn too
                            Trust from word go
                            To trust me I'd be open and honest
                  Empathy: put yourself in their position
                            Trying to get patient to talk back
  Skills required to form TR Patient personal
                  Different approaches support
                  Different approaches require 2 way reassuring
                  different skills conversation encouraging
                  different nursing styles self confidence
                  acquire different skills down to your
                  Non-threatening confidence
                  Duty of care is to encourage
                  Competence

Relaxed and calm approach
Not to be confrontational
Female nurses are able to
get around male patients
let them know
talk normally
hand gestures

Nursing is providing a service
    a service aiming for service satisfaction
        different services
        work as a team
        working with colleagues
        mightn't converse with a patient
        Responsibility: to get tasks done
            More responsibility more authority
            You're in charge
            Would affect my TR
            Responsible for own actions
        Same nurse
        Role
        Hospital not a nice experience
    Duty of care: providing care for those who can't provide it for themselves
        Role changes with experience
        When it's quieter on the ward

Experience Learn through practice
        Experience: learn over time
        Choice of therapies
            Colleagues step in
        Learn when a student
        All the experience
        Learn skills through experience
        My own framework
        Never learn from a book
        Students can't say too much in case say wrong thing
        Learn so many things from different colleagues
        Reading the situation
        It's my experience
        Watching colleagues
        I think it's just practice

Take the situation as I see it
You'd know the next time

Intuitive nature of TR learned
    Conscious effort versus use intuition
    Naturally performed your own intuition
                Your gut instinct
                  Never the same situation
                  Words I'd use
                  In my head
                  I would have known anyway
                  If you have intuition
                  Gut instinct
                  Go with the flow
                  Niggling you
                  I ride the waves

Helping or caring aspect causing stress if ventilating
    Of the TR you have help to give them
Quite distressed
                  They're distressed
                  They need help
                  Addresses you with their problem
                  Mightn't get anywhere
                  What is hoped to be achieved
                  Providing support for them
                  What kind of help I can provide
                  What I have to give
                  That will help them

Process of therapy Therapeutic factors Curative factors
                  Slow gradual change Kind of treatment
                  Answers questions put it into the TR
                  Caring medication
                  Engage the mind counselling
                  Compliance there for them
                  Advice care for people
                  Diffuse the situation talked down the person
                  Need some kind of treatment more independent
                  Not physical distance use that as a crutch
                  Patient opens up slowly regain independence

Adopt a different approach hospital environment
Giving something to the patients supportive network
Distraction Little niche of various patients
List of questions they're not going to open up
Know questions I want to ask

Professional aspects to Conduct yourself in a professional manner
  TRs have to be professional
                Pointing the finger
                Wouldn't be my place
                There is plenty of other staff for them
                What my role is
                Professional in work
                Professional person
                Professional all the time
                Stepping over the work
                Go through it with them
                Right decision
                Professional people
                A standard
                It is policy or procedure
                Right way to address somebody
                Cycle of treatment
                Dependent on nursing staff
                Supportive role of the nurse
                It is a more professional kind of relationship

Providing information On the level
to patients give them options
                give answers to questions
                give to the patient
                I've seen research on it
                Pinpoint
                I leave the issues

Impact of personal I don't bring it home with me
  life on the TR problems/involvement left at work
                less involved
                never bring problems into work
                have ups and downs

> human being at the end of the day
> only acting as somebody else
> straight living
> conduct self as in life
> never discuss private life
> not discuss problems
> my actions
> only natural
> it could be you or a member of your family
> they're human, you're human

Nature of the TR is *A situation*
    Dependent upon illness A low ebb
> Such a disturbed degree
> Opportunity
> Acute
> Buried so deep
> It is very frightening
> Pacing the floor
> Disruptive
> Anxious
> Not willing to engage
> Their mental state
> Lot of emotionally charged feelings
> Too distressed and upset
> Practically catatonic
> Stuperous state
> Psychotic depression
> Massive weight loss
> Tearful
> No appetite
> Pacing the floor

Conscious decision making Really have to stop and think
> Stand back
> Before you make a decision
> Think before you actually say something

Watch what you do or say

Appendix Ten

INTERVIEW NOTES

Participant 1- Date:28 – 4 – 04 Time: 3.30pm

Role
    Acute
Various   18 – Geriatric

Slower Approach

Intuition – prior to

Rapport – engage -   Two way   Relaxed
                                  Open   Calming

Personal -   safety security

Studying – school

Experience – Rogers

Responsibility –

Help – give help, treatment
Boundaries

Important – more in personal life

Distant

Emotionally charged – same rapport

Different in different circumstances.

Skills – Normally –
Layman's Language

Reassurance
Reward – Encourage
Responsibility
Praise

Open – Closeness

Intuition – Socialization
Gut instinct

Duty of Care

Noise
People looking in

Conversation – confides

Trust – Rapport

Participant 2- Date: 5-5-04 Time: 3.15pm

Acute – Role Various

TR – Getting to know patients
Time

Watch other nurses –
                Differences experience

Appendix Ten

Lesson the problem

Training read counseling skills role play

Respect – confidentiality – non-biased

Job to do – expecting help. Health professions – rules – problems opinions respected.

Stop and think.

Introduce –
Explain – ask questions

Reassurance Time

Understanding – thinking feeling

Skills – clear – tone voice

Rationale – open question

Looking at other nurses

Attitudes – non-judgmental

- re – attitudes/personalities

Continuity of care

Responding – independent – prompting

Scales – mood thoughts

Like – expand – honesty

Informed consent
Response – lye – genuineness

Participant 3- Date: 6-5-04 Time: 3.00pm

Care – limited – answerable to doctors

Therapy used – personal level.

Medical decision undermining nursing role.

16 – Geriatric

Professional build up balance friendly control and discipline

Distance – Trust
Confidential Non judgmental – personal issues

Classroom – learn properly
Mistakes – good? bad?

Level – impersonal approach
Rapport
    Experience – socialization

Love – different – bond
Different approach – things in common
Goal

Professionalism again – job

Giving care – more one sided relationship
Altruistic

Boundaries

Limitations – Relaxed

Codes of Practice

Friendly – not for granted – stigma

Continuity of Care – staffing levels

Set questions – suicide questions

Temporary admissions –

Personal – suicide

Friendly – professional. Shake not hug.

Codes – dress policies

On ward – mistakes – socialization

Watch other nurses – adapt it to own needs

Tool base -   Reachable
              Approachable

Confides

Similarities – one way
Time limiting. Goal

Participant 4- Date: 11-5-04 Time: 4.00pm

Help get better – care

Pre hostel – long term

One way – help *in crisis*

Trust you – confidence – realism
See when need help

Intuition – Experience - * Sixth sense

In classroom – heard what should do!

See relationships.

Watching – through the years.

Apprenticeship.

Detached – your problems

Obliged – in position to help
Here for money

Your experiences – keep it one way – opinions
Burden them with your issues

Personal space – touch

Artificial – personality betrayed

Primary nursing – personality clashes

Get to know the client – talk. Observe.
Joking

Basic – perceive – scientific debate

Observational – <u>open</u> – <u>approachable</u>
Authoritative
Non judgmental –
Time – making beds –
Medication

College – languages. Not nursing skills

Shouldn't but do.
Non judgmental – distance
Right in *middle*

You feel they can come to you
Perception – approachable

Trust – trust – open – dependence – independence
Sharing

                              Trust

Observation – non-verbal
Openness

Can't learn – Intuitive

Past experience

Participant 5- Date: 9-6-04 Time: 3.30pm

Team – MDT –

On hand – being there

Focal – View liaise more contact
In awe
Medium Support –
Skills
Link up – draw somebody out. Better rapport

Rapport – trust. Parent

TR – understanding trust help liaise link
Confident – best interests

- Listen to – *in the firing line*
- Block – research – on wards – other staff

In work frame of mind
Step into different – professional

Personally Involved	Intimacy - Boundary
No No	Time

Duty of care. Vulnerable – advocate

Trained – nurses interest – who are you?

First – introduce – word of comfort
Reassurance

Joke – normalizing

Stigma

Trial and error – honesty and trust

First impression – friendly face

Revolving door – frustrating

Joke – humor – straight-laced – need to know

Comfortable in your presence

Advocate -   spending time
         Direct contact
Overwhelming. Informative

Contentment – comforting to have a nurse.

Participant 6- Date: 5-7-04 Time: 4.00pm

Liaison – doctor – nurse – level
Education – symptom – services

Catchment – socio economic –

Acutely ill –
Action – no formal diagnosis

TR – student? – both people?

Personal skills – tool - talk
   Listen – action

Experience – skill –

Daily activities – hit – miss

Use of knowledge – similarities Code

Professional distance – boundaries
Differently – emotional

Professional requirements – touch –

Drink – therapeutic setting – objective
Paid

Trust – patient requirement – dementia
Intuition – care plan – broad strokes
Assessments
No
Language – short sentences – simple words
Lead – patient
Empathy – skills – knowledge of illness
Cures

Groups –
Non-threatening open eye contact
Dementia

Hypersensitive

Formal plan – relate

Child – open – job specific – interaction

Opinion – attitudes

Non-judgmental – 2-way process

Interaction – dementia – mood lifts

Information – knowledge

Appendix Eleven

Audit trail

It is vital to make explicit decisions made during research process to enable consistency and transparency in the research process. The decision or audit trail for this study began by identifying the research question.

Questions Asked During the Decisions Made in Relation to the Research Process Questions

Why choose the research question?

The notion that informs this study and what makes it a significant research endeavor is the questioning of the fundamental role of psychiatric nurses. Namely if psychiatric nurses claim to form therapeutic relationships with patients, are they doing this knowingly, with a complete understanding of why, how and when these relationships are formed?

Why review the literature?

The literature review in grounded theory provides context to concepts and an awareness of gaps in the literature. Grounded theorists maintain a second literature review is required to link a priori knowledge and new theory or evidence (Hutchinson and Wilson, 2001).

Why choose the Naturalistic paradigm?

Naturalistic inquiry is the most appropriate approach to use in this study. The research question is what determines the method of research adopted and in this case the research question seeks to ascertain what psychiatric nurses perceive to be the constituents of the therapeutic relationship. Naturalistic inquiry accepts that there are many perceptions of what constitutes reality and the objective of this study is to explore perceptions of psychiatric nurses' perceptions of what forms the relationship between nurse and patient and what makes this relationship therapeutic.

How does grounded theory 'fit'?

Strauss and Corbin (1990) describe one the purposes of research is to guide practitioners' practices and to develop a basic knowledge. In this study the objective is to form a theory relating to constituents of the therapeutic relationship to inform professional psychiatric nursing practice. Building theory implies interpreting data that must be conceptualised and the concepts related to a view of reality.

What rationale for the chosen sample?

Having located the research question and identified research methods it is incumbent upon the researcher to define and access a sample. The sample for this study was a purposive sample of six psychiatric nurses. The rationale for Purposive sampling as opposed to any other form of sampling lies with the selected methodology. Grounded theory requires information to be obtained from a particular research population this population must how the information required. In this study the information required is located in psychiatric nurses who are post qualification between two and ten years.

Rationale for inclusion criteria?

The sample nurses were generic psychiatric nurses with no post registration training in counseling or related courses that could bias the data towards a counseling orientation. The research refers to psychiatric nurses' perceptions of the constituents of the therapeutic relationship that could be biased by extra training in counseling. Psychiatric nurses qualified between two and ten years.

With who was access negotiated?

Access to conduct the research was negotiated with a number of gatekeepers before the commencement of the study. These gatekeepers included the Director of Psychiatric Nursing Services, the Programme Manager, Ward Managers and the Individual nurses involved in the study. The researcher must seek to gain ethical approval to conduct the study from appropriate authorities.

How was the sample selected?

The Assistant Director of Nursing department was requested to furnish me with a list of names of nurses who fulfill the inclusion criteria. Nurses who met the inclusion criteria were selected from the list. The nurses who were selected to participate were requested to on the basis of the research question and the notion that they hold the required answers to this research question.

Why use semi-structured depth interviews?

Individual semi-structured interviews were chosen as a method of data collection. This method enabled a flexible approach to data collection and fits with grounded theory methodology (Morse and Field, 1985). More structured data collection methods would not be consistent with a grounded theory approach, as it would not allow the participants the opportunity to expand on their responses to the questions posed in the interview.

Why include an interview guide?

It comprised open questions and was used as a reference to prompt me during the interviews, as I am a novice researcher. It was sufficiently structured to allow me to deviate from the guide to explore the participants' world and to expand on important information that was emerging.

Why topics were included in the guide?

An interview guide was developed informed by the available literature and upon my own experiences as a psychiatric nurse.

Why devise a GANT chart?

A GANT chart outlines the sequence of events through the research process. This chart enabled me to remain focused on the issue of time and provided deadlines for various phases of the research.

Why conduct a pilot study?

In this investigation the objective of the pilot study will be to test the interview schedule and to ascertain whether the answers given and the data collected are appropriate to answer the research question.

What was learned from the pilot study?

The pilot interview was a useful exercise in this particular study, to identify repetitions in the original interview guide that where altered in subsequent interviews. I also learned that the timing of the interview was good and gave sufficient scope to explore areas as they emerged from the participants.

Why interview in situ?

The presenting phenomena are studied in their own context and are specific to circumstance. Naturalistic inquiry seeks to gain knowledge through understanding how individuals interpret their own circumstances (Treacy and Hyde, 1999). To this end data are collected by interviewing and observing participants in situ.

How was transcribing performed?

When the data was transcribed the tapes were played simultaneously to readings the transcripts to verify the content as correct. These transcripts were copied and stored in a locked draw; the original documents were used for analysis.

Informed consent?

Prior to the interview commencing I sought permission to record the interview and to take notes as required, each participant granted this. I reassured each participant of the commitment to maintain confidentiality and anonymity prior to each interview.

What was the analytical process?

When the interviews were transcribed any names reference to names or places was erased or references were coded to maintain anonymity. The constant comparative method was achieved in this study by constantly returning to the data, moving between open coding and axial coding, comparing codes with categories, categories with sub-categories and constantly cycling between these areas. This constant cycling allowed me to engage fully with the emerging data and to provide concepts to explain phenomenon.

Why include memos?

To induce a grounded theory the analysis of data must be elicited at a theoretical level. Memos were part of this procedure to apply principles of constant comparative analysis, in the form of index cards, journal recordings or on a computer to establish connections between the data.

How did I arrive at the categories?

The process of amalgamating sub-categories and codes was commenced tentatively at the beginning of the analysis. The process as stated is a constant comparative method and referring to the codes sub-categories and memos, I began to link sub-categories with concepts or ideas that encapsulated the amalgamated sub-categories and codes. The categories that were produced encapsulated the open codes represented more abstract definitions of the sub-categories. Sub-categories were allocated to categories as they emerged and seemed to describe the resultant data.

Is the study rigorous?

Sandelowski (1986) describes four aspects of trustworthiness promoting rigor within the naturalistic paradigm. These four criteria refer to credibility, applicability, consistency and confirmability. These four principles of trustworthiness have been upheld throughout the research process.

What ethical considerations were made?

Confidentiality must be considered in relation to ethical considerations; it is based on the right to anonymity and linked to the ethical principle of the respect of person. Informed consent must be given in the light of the following and may be withdrawn at any stage of the research process. Ethical approval to conduct the study was sought from the Director of Nursing and Regional Manager.

How did I check confirmability?

Confirmability is reinforced in this study by the production of research notes made during each interview and the transparency of the decision trail. Notes were taken during each interview to assist in the data collection process and to assist in the data analysis.

Appendix Twelve

Feedback from psychiatric nurses and participants
regarding the findings of the study

John (pseudonym)- Community Mental Health Nurse- 25 years psychiatric nursing experience.

I clearly identify with the findings of the study, particularly in relation to

- The professional relationship aspect of the findings.
- Individual needs of patient care

It was interesting to identify the issue of temporary admission patients and the difficulties identified in relation to forming relationships. As a CMHN I am a bit removed from that scenario.

What I can relate to when in contact with staff on the wards is how limited numbers of staff and the continuity of staff effects the development of the therapeutic relationship.

One interesting point that I would have been aware of but possibly not the degree emphasized in the study is the effect my practice has on more inexperienced psychiatric nurses.

The final aspect taken from the study was the notion of genuineness; it wasn't there 20 years ago. Nurses today have a far more educative role than when I trained.

Peter (pseudonym)- Community Mental Health Nurse (Psychiatry of the old aged)- 25 years experience as a psychiatric nurse.

I haven't anything to add to your findings, I think it's excellent and a good representation of my practice as a psychiatric nurse.

INDEX

A

accountability, 47
accuracy, 34
acute, xi, xv, 16, 17, 47, 76
administrative, 93
agent, xi, 36, 52
agents, x, 5, 70
aid, 58
animals, 61
anxiety, 9, 60
appendix, 23, 26, 28, 31, 33, 34, 35, 36
appetite, 102
application, 7, 14, 29, 54, 73, 74, 77, 79
assessment, xvi, 18, 78, 79
assignment, 72
assumptions, xiii, 8, 14, 19, 22, 30, 68
asylum, 3, 17
attitudes, xvi, 4, 5, 6, 7, 8, 9, 18, 26, 40, 46, 48, 62, 63, 64, 65, 67, 74, 78, 79, 86, 105, 111
authenticity, 19
authority, xi, 99
awareness, vii, 2, 6, 10, 12, 70, 113

B

bad day, 48
barrier, 63
batteries, 28
behavior, 1, 12, 43, 49, 54, 62, 65
behaviours, 8
beliefs, xiii, 8
beneficial effect, 73
benefits, 36, 89
bias, 23, 39, 114
binding, 93
bonds, 13
burnout, 64

C

catalyst, x, 7
catatonic, 102
categorization, 13
category a, 51
category d, 45, 46, 47, 48, 49, 50, 51, 52, 53, 54, 55, 57, 61, 62
classroom, 107
clients, 3, 12, 13, 43, 45, 56
clinician, 5
closure, 26, 84
codes, 23, 26, 30, 31, 32, 33, 44, 46, 52, 53, 68, 83, 84, 116
coding, 30, 31, 32, 33, 36, 75, 83, 84, 91, 116
coherence, 54
cohort, 45

communication, 1, 2, 3, 5, 11, 61, 72
community, 17, 33, 77
competence, x, 10, 60, 73, 79
complexity, x, 74
components, ix, xi, xiii, 4, 8, 10, 15, 68, 73, 79
comprehension, vii
conception, 7, 74, 93
conceptualizations, vii, xiii, 3, 5, 6
conditioning, 10, 70
confidence, 28, 36, 50, 98, 107
confidentiality, 27, 36, 50, 105, 116
conflict, 44, 51
confusion, 48, 62
consciousness, 19
consensus, 15, 79
consent, 25, 36, 88, 89, 105, 116, 117
constraints, 23, 25, 33, 57
construction, 20
constructionism, 21
constructionist, 20
continuity, 44, 119
contracts, 57, 72
control, xii, 29, 43, 44, 51, 106
counseling, xiv, 1, 2, 11, 23, 24, 39, 57, 72, 105, 114
covering, 2, 84
crack, 59
cracking, 60
credibility, 34, 117
criticism, 12
cues, 54
cultural practices, xii
culture, xii, xvi, 17, 20
curiosity, 53, 70
curriculum, 24, 40, 53, 79
cyclical process, 28
cycling, 30, 116

D

data analysis, 19, 21, 35, 37, 38, 117

data collection, 2, 12, 14, 19, 25, 26, 27, 30, 34, 35, 37, 75, 115, 117
data set, 13
decision making, 41, 57, 60, 102
decisions, 23, 32, 34, 44, 49, 51, 54, 65, 113
definition, 4, 5, 70
delivery, x, 45, 61, 69
dementia, 111, 112
depressed, 46
depression, 102
detachment, 63
developmental factors, 10
developmental psychology, 74
dichotomy, 44, 69
dignity, 58
disability, 49, 52
discipline, x, xii, 4, 34, 39, 43, 46, 51, 55, 106
disclosure, 36
discomfort, 87
discourse, 15, 79
Discovery, 78, 83, 84
diseases, x
disorder, 46, 51, 52
distress, x, xii, 3, 73
diversity, 40, 41, 55, 74
division, 24
doctors, 45, 106
dominance, 3
double helix, 10, 13
duration, 25, 89
duties, 41, 53, 56, 60

E

echoing, 9
educators, 13
emerging issues, 28
emotional, 10, 50, 55, 62, 70, 87, 97, 111
emotions, 6, 48, 70
empathy, 7, 9, 74

empowered, 45, 75
empowerment, xii
encapsulated, 32, 116
encouragement, xii, 9
engagement, 10, 64
environment, 20, 22, 28, 49, 101
epistemological, 15, 80
epistemology, xii, xiii, 14, 19, 20
ethical principles, 35
ethics, 43
evolution, x, 22
exercise, 26, 73, 80, 115
existentialism, 8
exposure, 11, 24, 39, 54
extrapolation, 9
eye contact, 59, 111
eyes, 29, 35, 58

F

failure, 9, 40, 65, 67
fairness, 35
family, 5, 70, 102
fears, 9
feelings, 48, 59, 71, 87, 97, 102
flow, 33, 100
fluid, 47
free will, 98
freedom, 35

G

gauge, 64
generation, 1, 30
Geneva, xvi
Gestalt, 78
gestures, 99
grounding, 30
groups, 31
growth, 7, 8
gut, 54, 71, 100

H

handling, 48
harm, 35
healing, xi, xii, xvi, 6, 13, 17
health, 2, 4, 5, 10, 11, 72, 73, 75
health care, 5
heart, 17, 58, 71
helix, 10, 13
highlighted words, 31
honesty, 105, 110
hospital, 23, 47, 55, 61, 101
human, x, xii, 1, 4, 12, 14, 15, 22, 46, 48, 54, 61, 65, 72, 73, 78, 80, 102
human behavior, 1, 62
human experience, x, 4, 12, 14, 15, 72, 80
human nature, 65
humanism, xi
humanity, 5, 70
hygiene, 98
hypothesis, 30

I

identification, xiii, xiv, 6, 7, 67, 69, 74
identity, 3
ideology, 16
illumination, 83
implementation, 1
in situ, 20, 49, 116
in vivo, 31, 83
inclusion, 23, 24, 39, 114
independence, 52, 100, 109
indication, 52
individuality, 74
informed consent, 25, 36, 88, 89
initiation, 5, 70
inmates, x, 3, 4
insecurity, 15, 80
insight, 48
instinct, 54, 71, 100, 104

interaction, xv, 14, 16, 18, 22, 33, 54, 76, 111
interactions, 8, 20, 22, 33, 71
interpersonal communication, 3
interpersonal relations, xii, xiii, 2, 6, 11, 15, 17, 69, 79
interpersonal relationships, xii, xiii, 2, 6, 15, 69, 79
interpersonal skills, ix, xii, 1, 3, 7, 14, 26, 56, 57, 73, 74, 79
intervention, xii, xiv, 8, 9, 41, 50, 55, 68, 70, 73, 98
interview, 25, 26, 27, 28, 29, 31, 35, 87, 115, 116, 117
interviews, vii, 11, 12, 13, 25, 26, 27, 28, 29, 31, 34, 65, 75, 83, 87, 89, 115, 116
intrinsic, 53
intuition, 8, 54, 55, 71, 100
Ireland, 39
isolation, 5, 70

J

job satisfaction, 64
jobs, 57
judge, 64
judgment, xi, 58
Jun, 91
justification, xii, 36

K

Keynes, 37

L

language, 22, 47
laser, 29
laughter, 8
law, 88
laws, 20

learning, vii, 17, 22, 40, 41, 45, 53, 54, 55, 57, 70, 71, 77, 79
life experiences, x, 49
lifestyle changes, 51
lifetime, 65
limitations, 1, 33, 40
Lincoln, 19, 35, 37
linear, xii, 1, 20
links, 32, 98
listening, 8, 9, 26, 28, 58, 73
London, xv, 16, 17, 18, 37, 38, 76, 77, 78
love, 46

M

maintenance, 5, 36, 72
maladaptive, 6, 69
management, ix, 3, 93
manic, 47
manipulation, 20
manpower, ix, 26
mass media, 5, 70
matrix, 5, 8, 33, 40
meanings, 13, 22
measurement, 7, 20, 75, 80
media, 5, 59, 70
medication, 52, 100
Medline, 2
mental health, x, xi, xii, xv, 2, 3, 5, 10, 11, 16, 17, 18, 52, 75, 77, 78
mental illness, xi
mental state, 102
mentor, xv, 77
metaphors, 9
models, 6
modern society, xii
money, 108
mood, 105, 112
moral development, 73
morality, 72
morals, 43, 49
movement, 52, 86

mutual respect, 63

N

narratives, 13
natural, x, xi, 12, 43, 53, 61, 65, 70, 102
natural science, x
natural sciences, x
nature of time, 40
negotiation, 19, 25
network, 101
New York, 16, 17, 18, 37, 38, 76, 77
NK, 37
normal, 52
normalization, 52
norms, xi

O

objective reality, 20
objectivity, 6
observations, xi, 83
occupational, xvi, 77
old age, 120
openness, 56
orientation, 23, 114

P

Pacific, 16
paradigm shift, xii
participant observation, 71
partnership, 6, 8, 10, 15
patient care, xii, 3, 71, 119
patients, x, xii, xiii, xiv, 3, 5, 7, 8, 17, 43, 44, 45, 46, 47, 48, 49, 51, 52, 53, 56, 57, 58, 59, 60, 61, 62, 63, 64, 65, 68, 69, 72, 73, 74, 76, 85, 99, 101, 104, 113, 119
peer, 17, 77
perception, xv, 3, 65, 77

perceptions, 9, 11, 13, 15, 17, 19, 21, 22, 23, 28, 29, 39, 40, 50, 51, 67, 75, 80, 87, 113, 114
personal history, 64
personal life, 41, 47, 48, 49, 103
personality, xiii, 41, 43, 45, 46, 51, 62, 63, 64, 72, 73, 108
personality differences, 51, 63, 64
personality disorder, 43
personality traits, xiii, 46, 63
persuasion, 10, 70
phenomenology, 20
Philadelphia, xvi, 18, 38
philosophical, xiii, 14, 37, 38, 72
philosophy, xi, 7, 22, 72
pilot study, 26, 115
play, 44, 51, 105
pluralistic, 17, 75, 77
politics, 33
population, 24, 35, 75, 114
positivism, xii
positivist, xii, 6, 15, 20, 80
postmodernism, 37
printing, 93
prior knowledge, 29
privacy, 97
private, 48, 102
production, 35, 117
professional development, 64, 73
professionalism, 62
professionalization, xiv
professions, 105
property, iv, 33, 49
psyche, x, 9
psychiatric patients, xiv
psychiatrists, xi
psychological illnesses, 48
psychology, 2, 73
psychotherapeutic, xi, 16
psychotherapy, xiv, 5, 13, 17, 57, 77
psychotic, 46
public domain, 36

Q

qualitative research, xii, 16, 18, 37, 38, 66, 78
quantitative research, 38
questioning, xiv, 8, 9, 33, 73, 113

R

range, 9, 36
reading, 2, 91
realism, 107
reality, vii, 1, 10, 19, 20, 21, 22, 30, 39, 70, 113, 114
recall, 12
recognition, 73
recovery, 52, 97
reflection, xv, 10, 13, 15, 16, 70, 72, 76, 80
reforms, xvi, 77
regulations, 33
relevance, 2
repetitions, 26, 115
reproduction, 53
research design, xv, 11, 26
Reynolds, 16, 18
rhetoric, 4
risks, 36, 87, 89
role conflict, 36, 40

S

safety, 58, 98, 103
sample, 23, 24, 25, 27, 32, 35, 39, 75, 114
sampling, 19, 24, 25, 83, 114
satisfaction, 64, 99
saturation, 23, 25
Schizophrenia, xv, 17, 77
school, 45, 53, 103
search, xv, 1, 2, 3, 27
searching, 27
second party, 9
secret, 36
secrets, 9
security, 58, 98, 103
self-awareness, 6, 10, 70
self-discovery, 8
semi-structured interviews, 27, 65, 115
sensitivity, xv, 33, 66
sentences, 30, 61, 111
separate identities, 71
services, 40, 99, 110
shape, 13, 22, 46, 68
shaping, xiii, 71
sharing, 12, 50, 69
skills, vii, ix, xii, 1, 3, 4, 7, 8, 9, 11, 14, 16, 17, 18, 26, 38, 40, 48, 54, 55, 56, 57, 61, 63, 65, 67, 71, 72, 73, 74, 76, 78, 79, 86, 98, 99, 105, 108, 111
skills training, 11
social life, 22
social sciences, 19, 36
socialisation, xvi, 22, 77, 98
socialization, xiii, 4, 5, 8, 53, 54, 70, 71, 106, 107
sociological, 33, 47, 75
sorting, 97
sounds, 8, 27
spectrum, x
speech, 18, 31
spiritual, 5, 6, 70
spontaneity, 7, 80
spouse, 4, 41
staffing, 44, 107
stages, 2, 5, 35, 72
standards, 54
stigma, 106
strategies, 16, 37
stress, 60, 73, 87, 100
strokes, 111
students, 37, 57, 68
subjective, ix, 5, 6, 12, 69
subjective experience, 5, 6, 12, 70
suffering, xi, 61
suicide, 107

supervision, 11
symbolic, 21, 22
symbols, 14, 20, 22
symptom, 110

T

target population, 24
teaching, 73
telephone, 24, 93
tenants, 26
tension, 8, 10, 60, 70
therapeutic approaches, 18
therapeutic change, x, 75, 86
therapeutic interventions, 43
therapeutic process, 8, 10, 15, 52, 79
therapeutic relationship, vii, ix, x, xi, xii, xiii, xiv, 1, 2, 3, 4, 5, 6, 7, 8, 9, 10, 11, 12, 13, 14, 15, 17, 18, 19, 21, 22, 23, 24, 26, 28, 29, 33, 39, 40, 41, 44, 45, 46, 47, 48, 49, 50, 51, 52, 53, 54, 55, 56, 57, 58, 59, 60, 62, 63, 64, 65, 67, 68, 69, 70, 71, 72, 73, 74, 76, 77, 78, 79, 80, 85, 86, 87, 89, 95, 113, 114, 119
therapists, 8, 12, 13
therapy, 2, 4, 5, 7, 10, 12, 13, 40, 41, 44, 47, 50, 52, 65, 67, 68, 69, 70, 74, 76, 100
thinking, 105
threatening, 98, 111
threshold, 24, 39
time constraints, 23, 25, 33, 57
time consuming, 28, 68
time frame, 32, 75
timetable, 93
timing, 26, 55, 115
tradition, x, 14
training, viii, 7, 11, 17, 23, 24, 39, 74, 114
transcript, 28, 31
transcripts, 25, 29, 30, 31, 116
transfer, 28
transition, xv, 3, 77
transparency, 9, 34, 35, 113, 117
travel, 13, 93
trust, xiii, 56, 57, 58, 59, 62, 74, 97, 98, 109, 110
trustworthiness, 34, 117
two-way, 75

U

unconditional positive regard, 9, 45
United States, 3
universal law, 20
unstructured interviews, 11, 13

V

validation, 34
values, xii, xiii
variables, 8, 27, 68
variance, 65, 73
variation, 32, 84
ventilation, 6, 9, 70, 73
verbalizations, 9
voice, 105

W

weight loss, 102
welfare, 72
well-being, 73
workers, 75
workload, 41
writing, 11, 56